A Cup of Tea on the Commode

My Multi-Tasking Adventures of Caring for Mom. And How I Survived to Tell the Tale.

LARGE PRINT EDITION

MARK STEVEN PORRO

North Carolina

Published in the United States by WriteLife Publishing (an imprint of Boutique of Quality Books Publishing Company, Inc.)
www.writelife.com

978-1-60808-294-0 (p)

Library of Congress Control Number: 2023933257

Book Design by Robin Krauss, www.bookformatters.com
Cover Design by Rebecca Lown, www.rebeccalowndesign.com

First editor: Andrea Vande Vorde
Second editor: Allison Itterly

Table of Contents

Dear Mom,

When I first moved out west to chase a dream, I wrote you a check for one million dollars along with a note: "This will be good one day." It never was. Though I experienced a few glimmers in Tinseltown, I never reached Hollywood's Holy Grail.

I hope what I gave you in your final years was more valuable than any amount I scribbled on that check. To me, it was priceless.

Love Always + then Some,
Mark. Yes, Mark with a k.

Genevieve's Vision

On a crisp, sunny spring morning, a merry band of well-dressed young children parades down Emmett Place, looking like they've just escaped Mass at Our Lady of Mount Carmel. Some skip, a few hopscotch, others weave, but most march in unison. The girls—hair in pigtails, ponytails, or pixie cuts—wear frilly white dresses, white lace socks, and patent-leather shoes. All carry flowers: a single stem or bouquet. The boys sport combed hair, dress pants, shiny black shoes, and starched white shirts neatly tucked in. Neckties are the norm, but a couple flaunt their individuality with bow ties. Each lad clutches a string anchoring a brightly colored balloon bobbing to and fro in the wind. The entire procession appears to be from an innocent time long past. As the parade rounds the cul-de-sac and approaches the second house from the end, each child turns, smiles, and waves toward a window on the first floor.

Inside, beyond the billowy curtains, propped up in a hospital bed, sits a frail, ninety-two-year-old Genevieve. Her kind eyes dance with delight as she waves to the children. It's uncertain whether she knows any of them, but that doesn't matter. What does is the long-absent and much-needed joy these children seem to bring her.

The last girl, holding a single daisy, stops and beckons Genevieve to join the parade. Amused and tempted, Genevieve chuckles for a moment before a wave of sadness erases her smile. Her eyes drift to an old black-and-white photo hanging on the front wall. In it sits a young girl with a soft brown bob that frames her cherubic face. She, too, wears a frilly white dress, white lace socks, and patent-leather shoes, and holds a posy of daisies.

CHAPTER 1

The Call

Okay, I'll just say so long now.
I'll be going. —Mom

M y mother's first attempt at dying, the first I knew of anyway, occurred February 5, 2011, nine days after her eighty-ninth birthday. I was working at my sister's design firm in East Grand Rapids, Michigan, making extra cash to keep my struggling Los Angeles snack-food business afloat. My carefree bachelor life made traveling back and forth between the Pacific coast and Lake Michigan easy, even for weeks at a time. I didn't have any children and few responsibilities outside of work. But everything changed when I received the call.

"Senior Connections said Mom just shut down. They didn't know what to do and told me to come get her," my brother Michael said.

I held my breath. Senior Connections was the activity center where my mother spent her weekdays.

Michael's voice trembled as he continued. "I carried Mom's limp body into the house and put her to bed. The doctor cut off all food, drink, and medications. Hospice is on the way."

My pulse spiked.

Hospice comes only when the end is inevitable. I had gone through this scenario fourteen years ago with my father. Two days later, he died.

I packed some clothes, my phone, my computer, and a dark suit, just in case. The next morning, I arrived at my childhood home in Ridgewood, New Jersey. Six of us grew up here. Two grew old, one died, and now maybe another. Except for a six-month sojourn after a fire in 1969, the Porros lived at 247 Emmett Place for over sixty years. Not only did it provide a roof over our heads but also a crew of furry pets: cats, dogs, mice, rats—yes, rats, but mostly cute ones—hamsters, guinea pigs, rabbits, and a stray squirrel or two. And, on one occasion, an opossum. Quite the method actor was he. But on *that* day, he took playing dead too far and his latest performance ended up being his last. As an asthmatic with all that dander floating around, it's remarkable that I too didn't die in that house. However, my fond memories in that charming, ivy-hugging stone-front colonial outnumbered all of those creatures combined. Even though I left thirty-six years ago when I was eighteen, I've always considered it home. And on any normal day, I'd sprint up those brick steps and burst through the front door without hesitation, but that day was different. That day I stopped, gathered myself, and took a deep breath before reaching for the tarnished brass handle.

Huddled in the hallway, Michael consoled the mother-daughter live-in team we hired three years ago to prepare meals, manage household duties, and keep Mom company. I referred to them as Tweedle Dee and Tweedle Dumb. Their ashen faces and palpable concern for my mother stopped me in my tracks.

"What happens to us if she dies?" Tweedle Dumb asked.

I bristled, more at myself for thinking they cared about anyone but themselves.

"You can stay as long as you need, no matter what," Michael said.

While I struggled to find comfort in Michael's words, the Tweedles did not. I shook my head, brushed past, and edged into Mom's room. She lay in bed, semicomatose and oblivious to the whirlwind of activity going on around her. Perched on a high-back chair, the Tweedles' black cat kept watch with his sinister golden eyes. I wondered if this was a sign of good luck or bad. Janice, the lead hospice nurse, patiently demonstrated proper care procedures to a reluctant student slumped in the corner. Tammy was a nurse's aide, who, for several months, bathed and dressed Mom in the mornings and readied her for bed at night. Though I hadn't heard much about Tammy before, her attitude spoke volumes.

I hadn't been home in several months. Weekly phone calls eased my guilt, but I had my reasons. In recent years, my well-mannered, well-behaved, happy-go-lucky mother—who often visited me in Hollywood to crash parties, meet celebrities, and dine at her favorite bistro,

Chin Chins—had morphed into a not-so-lovable character like Archie Bunker.

Her ranting, raving, and mood swings became the norm. I tolerated them behind closed doors, but not out in public. Two years ago, at her granddaughter's wedding, she moaned and groaned about every little thing, and loud enough for everyone to hear. To stifle further embarrassment, I parked her far from the garden ceremony where she at last found contentment with another curmudgeon who matched her gripe for gripe.

Last year, when I flew in from Los Angeles to celebrate her eighty-eighth birthday, years of well-disguised depression peaked. Her foul mood only let up at the Italian restaurant where she plummeted into a deep state of melancholy, making sure everyone had a miserable evening. That was the first time I cried over a plate of pasta, and for all the wrong reasons.

Mom had honed this selfish behavior in her seventies and perfected it in her eighties. Michael could stomach it. I could not. And I had no desire to spend any time with either of her personalities. But now that she could die at any moment, any excuse for my absence seemed petty and unforgivable. She was my mom, Archie Bunker or not.

I swallowed my shame until everyone, and the cat, had left the room. (I don't trust cats. I also have my reasons.) When I was finally alone, I sat on the edge of the bed and studied my mother. The drastic change—both kind and unkind— startled me. Here lay a shadow of her former self. She had endured fluctuating weight issues for most of my life. The steady diet of appetite-suppressing candies and an endless variety of rib-crushing girdles provided only short-term relief. With each faint breath, her thin, frail body barely moved. Her full, rosy cheeks were now pale and gaunt, her puffy eyes sunken and dark. They used to sparkle and yet also seemed to mask a distant sadness. And though closed, I suspect they still did. The lines circling her mouth were no longer subtle, marking the only sign of tension. Her long white hair was held in a tight bun by a purple scrunchie—surprising after decades of weekly perms that had once matched the tight white curls of her seventh and most loyal child, Zuri, a Bichon Frisé. Her diamond rings, her wedding band, and the tan lines they'd left behind were long gone. The sole survivor hugged a swollen finger that wouldn't relinquish it anytime soon, and for good reason. It held the birthstones of her six children. Her nails, as usual, were painted bright red, and they were one of the few things I saw that day that made me smile.

This was a different person from the one I'd last seen: softer, vulnerable. And, unfortunately, one determined not to rage against the dying of the light but to go gently into that good night.

But why? Why now?

Mom's life seemed worth living. She was in relatively good physical shape for her age. Her kids loved her, including me, despite my long absence. Eleven grandchildren produced five great-grandchildren with plenty more to welcome. She lived in our family home for five years, having returned after a four-year stint in assisted living that ended in a biting incident involving Zuri. Sunrise Senior Living's zero-tolerance policy sealed his fate. But a separation was out of the question because Mom and Zuri were emotionally tethered. Convinced that the powers that be had framed her dog, Mom declared as any good mom would, "If he goes, I go too." And back home sweet home they came.

In this rare instance, the family curse of never letting go of anything played in our favor. Despite years of neglect, Mom's vacant house was still fit to live in, making her return relatively easy. However, this homecoming came with a caveat. Since she could no longer manage on her own, we hired a support team to move in upstairs. And as Mom's stability and personal hygiene abilities declined, Tammy entered the fray. Michael lived close by, so he became the point man. He and my sister, Laurel, created a detailed care plan and schedule to keep everyone in sync. For five years, all seemed fine at 247 Emmett Place, but for one, clearly it was not.

CHAPTER 2

An Only Child

I don't like being alone. It's not pleasant. —Mom

Genevieve Mary Brennan was born on January 27, 1922. She and her parents, John and Wilhelmina, lived in Garden City, an upper middle-class Irish Catholic enclave on Long Island, New York. Tragedy came early to their happy home when Genevieve's only sibling, Georgina, had died at birth. Accepting her role as an only child, she developed her spunky, independent spirit early on. And though she relished being the center of attention, she didn't mind sharing it with her dachshund, Bitsy, who filled the sibling gap.

At eleven years old, tragedy struck again when William, Genevieve's favorite uncle, committed suicide. Confusion and grief over the death of another family member tightened her bond with her beloved Bitsy. As a teenager, Genevieve showed her true mettle. When a neighbor's dog attacked hers, she intervened, and that heroic move earned her one hundred stitches and deep, permanent scars. Her dream was to become a veterinarian, but that ended when her father told her, "That's a man's job." Still, her devotion to animals never waned.

John Brennan was a plant manager at Mergenthaler Linotype in Brooklyn. He enjoyed fishing and hunting, and shared his passion for both with his daughter. Though Genevieve never shot an animal, she did enjoy target practice with her Colt 22 Officers Model Long Rifle pistol. Since veterinary school was out, she chose vocational school after graduating from Sewanhaka High School, hoping to join her father in the printing business.

In her late teens and early twenties, Genevieve earned her keep as a hand model. She had movie-star looks, but her long natural nails became legendary. However, she knew that career would be fleeting at best, so she took a job at Doubleday Publishing, where she filled her days proofreading juicy novels while studying for her degree at night.

At twenty-three, her dream of working with her father came crashing down when tragedy struck again. John Brennan died of a cerebral hemorrhage at the age of fifty-four. He was a heavy smoker, called it a curse, and begged his daughter to never take up the nicotine habit. She never did. When her father died, Genevieve's relationship with her mother, which had never been particularly warm, turned contentious and remained so. The pain she suffered from losing her father and, in a sense, her mother, prompted her to erect emotional walls few would ever crack. Genevieve inherited her toughness from her father, who, on the night before he died, not wanting anyone's pity, waited until his guests went home before he crawled up the stairs on hands and knees to his bed. She got her selfishness and guilt-tripping from her mother. I've got a bit of both in me.

During the Second World War, she volunteered at a local United Service Organizations (USO) to support the war effort. There, she fell for a wounded soldier, who was several years her senior. But the romance soured when he expected Genevieve and her mother to take care of him instead of the other way around.

The self-sufficient, independent Genevieve saw no appeal in that arrangement and broke it off.

She remained single until 1947, when mutual friends introduced her to Noel Porro. He was an army veteran, a chemistry student, and a devout Catholic from nearby Floral Park. Noel took a shine to Genevieve and took her to a Columbia University football game. Not the most romantic first date, but it proved to be a winner. Less than a year after they cheered on his alma mater to victory, family and friends cheered on Noel and Genevieve as they walked down the aisle, but not before tragedy struck again. Wilhelmina Brennan died of a heart attack just six weeks before the July 17, 1948 nuptials.

The newlyweds moved into the Brennan home, where Bitsy still stood guard. She grew jealous of the new addition. One day it got the best of her, and she bit Noel. Fearing she'd bite the next new addition, baby Laurel, they said goodbye to Bitsy. In 1951, after receiving his master's degree in chemistry, Noel accepted a job at Trubek Laboratories, and the New Yorkers were New Jersey bound. The young family moved to the village of Ridgewood, which was tucked in the southwest corner of the most northeastern county in the state. There they made 247 Emmett Place their new home. Over the next ten years, they welcomed five more children: Michael, Caryl, David, myself (Mark), and Diane Claire (Deecy). As the family expanded, so did the house. Three bedrooms grew to four, then four grew to five.

Emmett Place, a dead end—but only to traffic—was apparently built on fertile ground. Many families did their best to catch up with the Porro sixpack, which made our quiet cul-de-sac quiet no more. At least not until long after dark, when we kids, exhausted from hours at play, reluctantly trudged to our respective homes only to recharge and start again bright and early the very next day. The Porros lived in the second-to-last house on the right, close to the center of activities. Oh, the fun we had there. Spud, stickball, hide-and-seek where a witch did the seeking. Laurel was the best and the scariest witch. "Ollie Ollie in come free" always brought welcome relief, knowing someone else fell under her wicked spell.

Having five children in her first seven years of marriage, and a sixth four years later, might have pleased the Catholic Church, but it had to be a shock to Genevieve. (Okay, not a total shock because it takes two.) But as an only child, she'd never experienced other little people, let alone six of them. Noel, on the other hand, grew up surrounded by his five siblings and several cousins. He didn't experience peace and quiet until he joined the army. However, Genevieve adapted to her new reality and even thrived as a mother of six.

CHAPTER 3

The Lone Wolf

Mom: Before I die, I need to divvy up everything.

Mark: Like what?

Mom: The house, all the—

Mark: Don't worry. You already gave the girls your rings.

David got your dad's diamond. I got your gun. So, if I choose, I can have them all.

Unlike Mom, I liked being alone. I was born on July 5, 1957, the fifth of six children. I had two older brothers and two older sisters. My baby sister did not come along until four years after me. Growing up with my five siblings, finding alone time was rare, but I cherished every minute I could steal away from the others. Some called me a Lone Wolf.

In my youth, I suffered from asthma. Mom told me I nearly died at two years old. I remember many things, even at two, but I guess I blocked out that near-death thing. A combination of corticosteroid injections, suppositories, inhalers, and pills kept me breathing and alive. Wheezing and gasping for air was no fun, but I did enjoy certain aspects of the disease. If an attack came in the middle of the night, Dad gave me piggyback rides in the dark. We traversed the living and dining rooms while I steered by tugging on his ears. Left, right. Right, left. My poor father kept this up until the medicine kicked in and I fell back asleep. I fought hard to stay awake because I never wanted those rides to end.

The weekly steroid injections that should have caused fear and anxiety did not, in my case. Other than the smell of rubbing alcohol, a slight pain, and a bit of soreness after, I looked forward to those extra-long needles, because with every jab I got a coupon for a giant ice cream cone. That's what I remember most. I can still taste it, though the cones could have been crispier. I don't know who came up with that idea, but it was simply brilliant.

No one was happier about having a little brother than David. He, two and a half years older, filled my formative years with a variety of torture tests, but offered no treats to lessen the pain. His menu included clamping a jumper cable on my nose, stretching Mom's rubber exercise band from the vestibule, through the living room, to the far edge of the dining room, and then letting go of his end. The full body welt left an indelible mark inside and out. He also gagged, hogtied, and suspended me from the ballet barre in the basement for several hours before Dad rescued me. But his crowning achievement was coaxing me into the tumble dryer, closing the door, and turning it on. I took several spins before he let me out. If I could have squeezed into the washing machine, I'm sure that would have been next.

Michael occasionally joined in on the fun. When they made me cry, I stuttered, which pleased them to no end. Every now and then my steroid injections gave me a sense of euphoria, which emboldened me. On those days, I challenged my brothers. "You will not make me cry." They, of course, jumped at the chance. After several failed attempts, they stuffed me inside a baby's crib and rolled me down the stairs. I cried but survived. The crib did not.

The mash-up of astronaut/spy training David and Michael doled out toughened me up and no doubt had something to do with me wanting a little test dummy of my own. When I was four years old, my mother left for the hospital to give birth to her sixth child.

I demanded, "If you don't bring me a baby brother, don't come back." Those words actually tumbled out of my four-year-old mouth.

When the car pulled into the driveway a few days later, I ran out to meet it. Mom rolled down the window and told me I had a baby sister. My heart sank, but after one look I said, "She's all right. We'll keep her."

Two years later, when Deecy snuck up behind me and cracked a glass bowl on my head, I wondered if I'd made the right decision.

At five years old, severe stomach pains doubled me over. Mom rushed me to the Valley Hospital. My mother suspected appendicitis. The doctor disagreed and sent me home with a pale-green, egg-shaped pill. Two hours later, the pain returned with a vengeance, and we went back to the ER. This time, the doctor ran the proper tests. Mom's intuition was right. Surgery was scheduled for the next day. The Jell-O, the Lassie planter gifted by my kindergarten class, and my new supercool four-inch scar almost made the pain worth it. Almost.

A combination of curiosity and necessity drove me at an early age to learn how to cook, do laundry, and sew by hand and on a Singer. Why a sewing machine? When clothes shopping, Mom gave me little choice. So I needed to make my skin-tight fashion-of-the-day alterations at home, under the cloak of darkness. I also cut my own hair for many years, which might explain my dating drought in high school.

Doing my own laundry presented a problem, a solution, and a missed opportunity. Synthetic fabrics dominated my wardrobe, thanks to Mom, which meant plenty of static electricity, especially in the winter. When I forgot to add fabric softener in the wash, I added some to a piece of terrycloth, let it dry, and tossed it in the dryer. It worked like a charm. This was years before dryer sheets hit the market. Oh, what could have been.

But my mind was elsewhere. In the eighth grade I decided to become an ophthalmologist.

I had no idea why, maybe because of my medical issues. But upon reflection I discovered the answer. My best friend at the time had an elevator in his house, heated sidewalks—no snow shoveling—and a limousine. His father was, you guessed it, an ophthalmologist. So, my goal was to go to medical school in order to have those same things. I visited only two colleges, Harvard when Laurel lived nearby, and Ohio State where she later majored in ballet. I chose Ohio State, not because of my grades or my SAT scores. They didn't matter to me, but apparently, they did to *you know who.*

I loved math and science but thanks to Mom, I also loved the arts. The thought of all those years of medical school without feeding my creative side caused me to reconsider my major. Lucky for me, Ohio State's College of Industrial Design married all three of my loves: math, science, and art. And lucky for me, they had one of the best programs in the country.

After graduation, I worked my butt off at a local design company for four and a half years before one of the best design firms in the country stole me away. But in 1984, I caught the acting bug and moved to Hollywood to chase a dream. Design continued to support me during my lean years in Tinseltown, and in between all my various business ventures.

CHAPTER 4

Mum's the Word

We said it was a heart attack. —Mom

At Grandma's house, I heard whispers of Adolf, a popular name in the first half of the twentieth century before *you know who*. But when seeking any details about who they were referring to, I heard the typical refrain of my parents' generation when dealing with uncomfortable subjects:

"Mum's the word."

In 1971, I met my uncle Adolf for the first and last time at his wake. He died of a cerebral hemorrhage after he fell at a Long Island Veteran's Hospital, his home ever since he was injured in World War II. Death wasn't totally new to me. By fourteen, I'd already experienced the loss of many pets. But this was the first time I had been face-to-face with a dead person, my father's older brother. Adolf didn't look much like Dad, especially in that waxy state, yet the family resemblance was clear. Seeing him in that coffin all but shattered my belief that my dad was immortal. If there was any order to these sorts of things, Dad was next.

Scanning the chapel, I noticed that nobody was crying. Quiet, respectful, but no one looked particularly sad. Everyone seemed to have a sense of relief. I didn't understand why. He was only fifty-nine and the first of his generation to die. Years later, Dad filled me in on a few scarce details about my mysterious uncle. During their teenage years, Adolf—the black sheep of the family—and the studious Noel had a falling out. Both went off to war. Adolf suffered a brain injury that left him permanently disabled, making an improbable truce all but impossible. What happened at the veteran's hospital during the last twenty-eight years of his life remains a mystery to this day.

Mum's the word.

Adolf's wake also marked my introduction to Aunt Claire's obsession: photographing the dead. Not just any dead, but dead relatives in their coffins. This macabre tradition was popular in the Victorian era, and Claire kept the custom alive deep into the twentieth century. She didn't take her memorial portraits behind closed doors; she did it out in the open for all to see.

After all mourners had paid their respects, Claire strolled up to the casket and fired off several shots with her handy Instamatic. The sudden bursts of bright light woke up the room and everyone in it. I was surprised Adolf didn't sit up and say, "Really, now you take my picture?"

Claire offered no apology but only a giggle as she scurried back to her seat. I'll chalk it up to the old adage, "We all grieve in our own way."

Weeks later, just when I got that image of my dead uncle out of my head, a four-by-six glossy arrived in the mail to haunt me all over again. It gave me the same queasy feeling as when my sister Caryl introduced me to her own obsession: picking scabs. Not just any scabs— *my* scabs while I slept. I caught her only once, but even that was once too many.

Aunt Claire continued to send me memento mori prints ever since. When my father died, I hoped she'd broken from tradition. No such luck.

If Only

My mother's uncle William never married, had no children, and lived with his mother until her death. As I write this, the irony is not lost on me because I, too, have never been married, have no children, and lived with my mother until . . .

Anyway, my great-uncle William had issues. Profound issues. I, on the other hand, am perfectly fine, thank you very much. Apparently, William couldn't come to terms with the loss of his mother, so he decided to leave this earth early, on his terms, perhaps comforted by the thought of reuniting with her in heaven. On second thought, a Catholic committing suicide is a mortal sin and therefore bound to spend eternity in hell. So, there's *that*.

As Mom told it, William set up a shotgun in his basement with a pulled string tied to the trigger. Just as he put the barrel into his mouth, the doorbell rang, and rang, and rang. For any number of reasons—losing his nerve, having concern for his loved ones, or the bloody mess he surely would have left behind—William aborted the mission and answered the door.

Genevieve, who was eleven years old at the time, bounced into his house. On that lovely warm afternoon, she came over to invite her favorite uncle to join her for an ice cream cone. He graciously declined. Though disappointed, she continued on her way, once again leaving him alone.

That was the last time Genevieve saw her uncle William. Her interruption may have caused him to lose his nerve but not his resolve. He was found in the kitchen with his head inside the gas oven. Death by asphyxiation. Sounds cliché now, but back in the 1930s it was a convenient, clean, and effective method to end your life. He left no suicide letter, so his rationale remained uncertain. While searching for clues, the police discovered William's shotgun set up in the basement. It appeared young Genevieve's visit prompted him to choose the less violent exit. So, there's *that*.

A year before William took his life, he'd built Genevieve a dollhouse, a replica of her childhood home. It had awnings on the outside. Curtains on the inside. A fireplace and chimney. Wallpapered walls. Carpeted floors. Tiny furniture in every room. Doors and windows inside and out that worked. Lamps that actually lit. It even had a doorbell that rang. He lined the perimeter with a variety of trees and shrubs. Woodworking skills are another thing Mom's uncle and I have in common. William's masterpiece found a new home in ours for many years, then in Caryl's and Carl's, where—after a sprucing up that thrilled Mom to no end—it entertained their three daughters for many more. Perhaps its constant presence made it easier for Mom to share his tragic story.

The specter of mental health was undoubtedly taboo back then and rarely discussed. Even today, the subject evokes a certain level of discomfort, if not utter shame. No one heard William's silent scream for help except perhaps his niece, who made that impromptu visit. If only he'd accepted her invitation on that fateful day. Could that simple gesture have made all the difference? Mom said she always regretted that she didn't insist he join her. A heavy and undeserved burden for her to carry all those years. Wishing things were different might be futile, but sometimes we can't resist the temptation to ask, "If only?"

We Said It Was a Heart Attack

In 1993, while Mom was visiting my sister Deecy and her newborn in Michigan, Mom suffered a major stroke. She had just turned seventy-one. Deecy called me with the disturbing news.

"She started mumbling in the car, and then the left side of her face just dropped."

I didn't want to believe it. My mom was invincible, one tough cookie. I needed to hear her voice. Deecy held the phone for her. A deep, gravely—definitely not my mother's voice—slurred, "Don't come, I'll be fine."

Another Porro refrain. No matter what the circumstances are, we don't like to burden others, even family. Other than the usual nicks and scrapes we incurred while dealing with life's adventures, the Porros had been fortunate. Mom's stroke was our family's first critical health crisis. Of course I would fly out to Michigan. My dad offered to join me from New Jersey, more out of duty, but since there was not much love left in their forty-five-year marriage,

I asked him not to come. He understood and stayed put. I caught a red-eye out of Los Angeles and arrived in Grand Rapids early the next morning.

Mom recently retired from her thirty-year proofreading career at *The Record*, New Jersey's largest newspaper. But for fun, she searched the "daily" for typos the computers often missed. Although both of my parents were spelling and grammar sticklers, Mom's eagle eye was the one I feared most. That seasoned skill would come in handy to gauge her current condition. I had recently designed an art gallery invitation for a new client. There was a typo on the printed piece that had been missed by fifteen people, including me. I took one of the invitations with me to Michigan.

When I entered her hospital room, Mom, not too surprised, greeted me with a droopy smile and that deep, gravely—definitely not my mother's—voice. "I told you not to come."

Fighting back tears, I kissed her forehead and said, "I know." After overcoming my initial shock, I handed her the invitation. She spotted the typo in no time. I smiled and said, "You're gonna be all right." When I told my client about it, he insisted on hiring her for all future projects. So much for retirement.

We had a lot of fun during Mom's hospital stay. She introduced me to her doctor, who she insisted looked like Dr. Greene from *ER*, and he certainly did. I asked him, "Should she be doing push-ups so soon after a stroke?"

"I did twenty," Mom mumbled without skipping a beat. "What's the big deal?"

He froze for an instant, then offered a surgical smile. When he realized our joking accelerated her recovery, the good doctor grew to appreciate the Porro Rehabilitation Technique.

Mom sailed through speech and physical therapy, and to everyone's surprise except mine, she returned home after just three weeks. I told you she was one tough cookie. Before discharging her from the hospital, the doctor conducted an exit interview that included questions about family history. When he asked about her mother's cause of death, Mom hesitated for a moment before muttering, "We said it was a heart attack."

The doctor's pencil skidded to a halt.

"I know. Wait, what do you mean, 'we said'?" I asked. She wavered. I pressed, but not too hard because she'd just had a stroke. "Mom?"

The doctor and I waited.

She bowed her head in shame, then blurted, "My mother killed herself." The doctor and I traded looks. Mom, in no hurry, continued. "She tacked up the carpets in the dining room and turned on the gas stove. I found her collapsed on the table. Father Joe told the police she died of a heart attack."

I sat in stunned silence. I knew little about my grandmother Wilhelmina other than she died before Mom was married. *But she killed herself? How do you respond to something like that?* My mind raced through my dating history in Hollywood. My Rolodex was filled with several women who possessed a vast array of mental disorders, including a psychic who suffered from dyslexia. She could only predict the past, and though she was incredibly accurate, she was as wacky as the rest.

But after racking my brain, the only comforting words I came up with were, "Mom, that is nothing to be ashamed of. Mental illness is a disease and needs to be treated like any other."

The doctor added his reassuring support, so I continued. "With Uncle William, and now your mother, suicide is a huge part of our family history. We need to know these things."

She nodded.

I don't know about my siblings, but I've had fleeting moments when I thought about ending it all. "Fleeting" being the keyword. However, this revelation about my mother's side of the family puts those and future thoughts in a whole new perspective.

I leaned in and asked, "Are there any other surprises?"

"Like what?" she asked.

"Like, are you really my mom? That kind of stuff." I held my breath.

She glared. "Yes, silly, of course."

I exhaled and sat back. Not that there's anything wrong with being adopted, but at that moment, I needed to know.

A few months later, after some prompting, I got the full story of my grandmother's suicide. In 1943, as Mom was leaving for work, her father waved goodbye from the upstairs bathroom window. Shortly after, her mother called and said, "Come home, something's wrong with

Daddy." When Mom returned home, she found her father lying in bed, already gone, and her mother was folding laundry, as if she were oblivious to the stark reality that was lying a few feet away. Wilhelmina appeared to be in denial and insisted, "He's fine. He's just sleeping."

On that day, Genevieve had lost her father to a heart attack and her mother to mental illness. As the disease advanced and Wilhelmina became more and more difficult to deal with, the doctors and Father Joe, the local parish priest, prescribed their best medicine: a mental institution. Twenty-three-year-old Genevieve, now in charge of her mother's well-being, yielded to the powers that be. Wilhelmina received electric shock therapy, which was less controversial in the 1940s. She felt betrayed by her only child. After she was released from the institution, Wilhelmina's bitterness grew until she could take it no more. She exacted her ultimate revenge by killing herself just weeks before her daughter's wedding.

After unleashing some choice words over her mother's dead body, Genevieve sought the aid of Father Joe and a neighbor. To protect her, they ripped down the carpets, aired out the house, and removed all evidence of Wilhelmina's unnatural death. Father Joe advised Genevieve to clear all joint bank accounts before calling the police because the banks would freeze the funds necessary for her upcoming nuptials. The family priest wielded much knowledge and influence in those days, but did he offer any investment advice?

Mum's the word.

CHAPTER 5

A Silent Scream

(I give Mom a hug. She wants no part of it.)
Mom: I want my teeth.
Me: I was trying to have a moment.
(She chuckles and points to the tray.)
Mom: My teeth.

The thought of ending her life must have crossed Mom's mind before. Depression ran on her side of the family, and as I learned after her stroke in 1993, self-destruction. Now in 2011, I sat on deathwatch and wondered if there was a specific event, or a series of events, that propelled my mother into what appeared to be a self-induced coma. Was she that unhappy, raging deep inside, but afraid to speak? Sure, she'd bitch and moan about little things. Social filters tend to fade with age. But Mom rarely expressed her true feelings and only when prompted. Was this one of those times? Was this a silent scream for help? Clues were everywhere if one cared to look. But evidently, no one dared because once seen, they couldn't be unseen.

I looked.

There were two printed photos taped to her bedroom wall that captured a few moments of Mom's eighty-ninth birthday party at Senior Connections nine days earlier. The proprietors made sure to celebrate every member's birthday because you never know how much time someone had.

In the top photo, Mom was clad in easy-on-easy-off stretchy clothes. She wore no makeup, not even her usual red lipstick. A cheap jeweled tiara crowned her unkempt hair. The wilted blue feather boa draped around her neck might have lightened everyone else's mood but failed to hide her pitiful smile. In the bottom photo, the staff, fellow octogenarians, and many of the East Coast Porros posed with Mom and her cake with flaming number eight and number nine candles. Her gaze to the camera screamed, "Get me out of here." And not just out of this place, but out of this life.

I looked.

Few remnants remained of Mom's existence beyond her bedroom threshold. Family photos, memorabilia, and knickknacks—previously displayed throughout her house—were now sequestered in her room. The coffee table I made in tenth grade was tucked in the corner. It had been a Christmas gift for my parents that had brought my mother to tears twice. The first was when I presented it, which at the time I didn't fully understand. I thought, *What, you think I'd make you a piece of junk?* The second time was when I pre-antiqued it while horsing around on my bongo board in the living room. That small dent might as well have been a stab to her heart. But antiqued or not, that table went on to win the top prize in the New Jersey State Industrial Arts competition. The craftsmanship must have surprised my dad as well, and it began the thaw between us. My quitting baseball and the Catholic Church in quick succession did not please my father, who was devoted to both. Dedication wasn't my problem. Dedication to *what* was.

Perhaps knowing how much that coffee table meant to Mom prompted the Tweedles to move it into the already-cramped space. Or perhaps they preferred their shabby-chic furniture they collected on junk days, which now dominated the house.

I looked.

The house screamed of neglect. Water leaks from the second-floor bathroom produced dripping holes in the ceilings below. The front door—rotting inside and out—made for unobstructed passage of winter's frigid winds. Old storm windows hung on for dear life to rusty frames. Cobwebs clung to every corner. Past and present junk engulfed the entire basement, attracting creatures who crawled while horrifying those who didn't. A hygienic bidet toilet seat with ill-fitted handrails might have kept Mom clean as a whistle, but it put any man's genitals in jeopardy. Though I must admit, the warm water jets drenching my nether regions were worth the risk, but I digress.

I looked.

Grain moths on uncontrolled flight patterns feasted on the Tweedles' buffet of snacks on display in unsealed boxes that were scattered across the kitchen counters and inside the cabinets.

I looked.

Mom must have resented all the changes going on in plain sight. Her welcoming home now repelled most visitors, including family. She spent less time with her loved ones, and more time with those who couldn't care less. Who could blame her for wanting to leave this life?

But for the moment, despite everything, I bit my tongue and camped out in the living room on the thirty-year-old twin-sized hide-a-bed and kept a close eye on everyone.

CHAPTER 6

You're Gonna Need a Bigger Fireplace

Save the wrapping paper. —Mom

On special occasions, Mom set the dining room table with her fine china and sterling silverware engraved with the Porro family crest and removed the plastic covers from the living room furniture. Only then could we kids take comfort knowing we wouldn't accidentally slide off our seats in the cool months or stick to them in the hot ones. This gave us another reason to love Thanksgiving, Christmas, and Easter Sunday.

Thanksgiving was a treat even with bellyaches thanks to the turkey, stuffing, and Mom's apple, cherry, and pumpkin pies. Bonnets, baked ham, and searching for Mom's lavish baskets overstuffed with candy sweetened our Easters. But only Christmas was an all-hands-on-deck family affair. Dad braved the blistering evening snow and a shaky ladder to hang garland and multicolored lights around our front door while the rest of us stayed warm by the fire listening to Bing Crosby and Nat King Cole croon Christmas carols. Mom and Laurel set up the Nativity scene on the mantel, keeping Baby Jesus off to the side. David and Caryl hung stockings emblazoned with our names—pets too—above the fireplace. Michael draped our fragrant Douglas fir with strings of lights with at least one nearly-impossible-to-find faulty bulb that threatened to disrupt our holiday cheer. Deecy and I decorated the tree with candy canes, tinsel, and ornaments, old and new. We crowned our masterpiece with an angel and prayed she'd watch over us, but I secretly prayed she'd bring me a bounty of gifts, never mind if I was naughty or nice.

After guzzling eggnog and stuffing ourselves silly with Mom's homemade cookies, the Porro kids placed our gifts under the tree and hustled off to bed to attempt the unthinkable: sleep the night before Christmas. But convinced we heard the clatter of reindeer hoofs on the roof made even a glimmer of hope impossible.

The morning, however, confirmed that what we heard was *what we heard*. Not only did Baby Jesus appear in the manger, but our meager offerings multiplied into a colorful mountain piled high and wide. The stockings were stuffed so full their seams screamed for merciful relief as they hung on for dear life to tiny brass hooks. Even with weary eyes, it was all a glorious sight to behold.

Our not-so-secret Santas spent the wee hours packing and wrapping to make our Christmas yet another one to remember. But there was one thing that stood in the way of us climbing up the gift mountain: church. We had to endure the torture to look but not touch until after the service. And once unleashed, it didn't take us long to rescue the stockings and tear into every package under the tree. Despite Mom's plea to save the wrapping paper, we left only shreds in our wake.

As our family grew, so did the Everest of gifts. This posed no problem for Mom, as it meant more shopping. That was our gift to her.

Even though the house could handle the ever-increasing numbers, the fireplace could not. The stockings spanned the entire face, two or more to a hook before spilling onto both sides. The sight inspired many comments from those who entered our festive home, but the one we heard most often was, "You're gonna need a bigger fireplace."

CHAPTER 7

Genevieve's Warehouse

Mom wakes, breathing heavy.
I rub her hand to comfort her.

Mom: You need socks?

Me: No.

Mom: Where are they?

Me: On my feet.

Mom: You have enough?

Me: Yes.

Mom: Good, 'cause I don't have any extras
to give you.

When I think of Mom, I think of shopping. We all do.

"Homemaker" might not have been her true calling, but she did her best. And when things got tough, she sought refuge not in pills, caffeine, or alcohol, but in shopping.

While Ridgewood offered several upscale clothing stores within walking distance, the real bargains were just a short drive away. The Garden State Plaza, the Fashion Center, the Paramus and Bergen Malls, as well as several New York City designer outlets—in less-than-designer locations—all beckoned. If and when jonesing for a sweet deal, one could score relief in minutes. It was all too tempting for Mom and her addiction.

To her credit, she excelled at finding bargains, in or out of season. However, winter steals bought in July were often too small by December. So those "no-return" super deals were anything but.

Raising a large family on his chemist salary caused Dad plenty of concern. Mom's habit only added to it. To ease financial tensions, she worked odd jobs by day and at Alexander's, a large retail store, at night. But like an alcoholic tending a bar, that proved to be too risky. Returning to proofreading full time at *The Record* seemed like the perfect solution. However, the graveyard shift at the paper left her days free to shop. That, combined with advance notice of upcoming sales, made it a mixed blessing at best.

We kids took turns struggling to keep up with Mom on her shopping marathons. She'd come home from work early in the morning, grab one or more of us, and off we went. She never seemed to tire. My aunt Flo accompanied her once, and only once. No one, not even me, could match her drive or stamina. I got bored early and often, more so as a teenager, though Mom tried her best to spark my waning interest.

"We have to go to this designer outlet. Ali MacGraw's ex-husband owns it."

I thought Ali was sexy, so I took the bait. No doubt my raging hormones influenced my decision. Mom drove through the Jersey swamplands—a.k.a. the resting place of many mobsters—to a dark, dank, derelict warehouse on the south side of Newark. There we met a suntanned, toupee-wearing, skinny man dressed in a tight paisley shirt and plaid polyester pants. Perhaps his fashion choices were the reason why Ali left him. Mom, however, insisted I follow the same recipe. I was the only kid who wore plaid and paisley *wonder fabrics* throughout middle and high school. I could have avoided that embarrassment if I'd stayed in Catholic school where uniforms were the norm. I was, however, the first seventh grader to wear bell-bottoms. Even though they were plaid, they still ratcheted up my "cool factor." So it wasn't all bad.

There were other times I accompanied Mom on her shopping sprees as more of a bodyguard. Mornings began innocently enough outside Pergament, a local home-improvement center. A cordial crowd of like-minded bargain hunters gathered hours before the store opened, making small talk while secretly salivating and jostling for position. But as soon as that sign flipped from Closed to Open and the door key turned, all hell broke loose. It was life or death for any man, woman, or child caught between the elbowers and the tramplers who were fighting for the 40 percent-off linoleum floor tiles. Mom relished these melees, evidenced by her regular participation. I did not. Leading the way like a fullback fending off all of Mom's would-be tacklers was no fun for me. She kept her cool and by doing so lost out on some of those do-or-die bargains. But we both survived. Me, battered and bruised yet happy in my role as protector, and she, excited and energized to try again another day.

If Mom had any self-control, she showed no signs of it at Christmas. The number of gifts she bought was, by any measure, absurd. Though we rarely, if ever, needed anything—except maybe something in a solid color or in a natural fabric—it didn't stop her from going a little nuts. And as grandchildren started popping out, she went even nuttier. Keeping track of who got what got complicated, making Christmas Day a guessing game for all. It was not unusual to see Mom snatch a gift from a child's hands and say, "That's not yours." Then she'd dash off to the back bedroom and return with a more suitable present.

Mom's shopping didn't appear to be a significant problem until unnecessary, un-wanted, and unopened purchases began to pile up. During a visit home in 1982, I joined her for lunch at one of her two favorite restaurants, which was located inside Lord & Taylor. Her other favorite restaurant, Kurth Cottage, was part of Valley Hospital. Both locations struck me as odd.

Having lunch out was a special treat for Mom but having it inside a large retail store was borderline dangerous. Of course she insisted on buying me something after we ate, and I always insisted she didn't. This only steeled her resolve.

"If you buy me anything, I will buy you the biggest stuffed animal in this store and announce to everybody that I am buying it for my shopaholic mother," I threatened. She called my bluff. I don't know if I was more angry or embarrassed when I jammed that gigantic gray gorilla into the backseat of her Acura. Mom was neither.

As the Porro children moved out and on with our lives, the impossible happened: Mom's shopping surged. When overstuffed rooms and closets on the first floor couldn't be overstuffed anymore, she took over the entire second floor. I christened her new storage space, "Genevieve's Warehouse."

Over the years, we kids all took stabs at thinning out the chaos. Laurel, the Purge Princess, blessed by having no emotional attachment to any of it, won the award for filling the most dumpsters. One time, after regretting starting the near-impossible task, I entertained placing an ad in *The Record*: "Fifty bucks for fifteen minutes. Grab all you can." Fearing Mom would not only proof the ad but answer it, I jettisoned that idea and continued clearing room after room. But creating space only gave Genevieve an excuse to fill it again . . . and fill it she did.

On rare occasions, a trip to Genevieve's Warehouse proved fruitful. I once caught my acoustically challenged father listening to a New York Yankees baseball game, unaffected by the ear-piercing volume and crackling static blaring from a ticking firebomb disguised as a clock radio. Its electric cord, cobbled together and wrapped in old cloth tape, posed a clear and present danger. He might not have cared, but I did. Knowing that parting with his junk, hazardous or not, would be difficult, I went straight to begging.

"Dad, please let me replace this. It's dangerous." To my surprise, he agreed. I bolted upstairs before he changed his mind to search the aisles of Genevieve's Warehouse for a replacement.

The sheer volume she'd accumulated be-tween each of my visits, though not surprising, still shocked, and nearly ignited my first asthma attack in decades. Though tempted to turn and run, I was on a mission. I squeezed past racks crammed with blouses, coats, and pants, many still enclosed in their original plastic. I sidestepped framed photos of strangers begging to be replaced by familiar faces, stacks of CDs never to be heard, and videos never to be watched. After stumbling over baskets overflowing with Beanie Babies and digging into yet another mountain of boxes, I found what I was looking for.

I hustled downstairs. "Dad, look what I found. A brand-spanking-new UL-listed clock radio." My enthusiasm fell on his already near-deaf ears. Undeterred, I removed the old one with its aluminum-foil-capped antenna, plugged in the new, tuned it to the now static-free game, and cranked up the volume to Dad level. He smiled when he heard that the Yanks were leading the Red Sox six to four in the eighth inning. I escaped with the old one and tossed it in the trash.

Later that night, I grew suspicious of my father's swift surrender. When I checked the trash can, the radio was gone. *Are you freakin' kidding me?*

Livid, I marched into his bedroom and demanded, "Where is it?" That stubborn son of a gun held his ground. The only person more stubborn than Dad was Mom, but I had the worst of both in me, and on that day, he'd met his match. I sat down and looked him straight in the eye.

"I'm trying to protect you and Mom. I can only do that if you let me. That radio is dangerous. If you plug that old one in and it starts a fire, and one or both of you gets hurt, or worse, do you know how guilty I'd feel?"

It worked like a charm. I found the firebomb wedged between way too many winter coats in the overstuffed front closet and wrestled it free. Taking no chances this time, I drove several miles away, one eye looking ahead, the other glued to the rearview mirror to make sure he wasn't tailing me in his brown VW Beetle. When I felt the coast was clear, I buried the radio in a gas station dumpster.

Mom continued to shop for me long after my "plaid phase." She bought shirts and pants I'd never wear inside my home, let alone out in public, until I begged her to stop. "Mom, we have different tastes."

Undaunted, she moved on to other things. When I mentioned my Bonsai trees kept dying in the California heat, she sent me a plastic one. I wasn't a fan of fake plants, so I hid it on my balcony where the Santa Ana winds swept it to its own untimely death three stories below. I took that as a sign. Neither of us ever bought another Bonsai.

The local economy suffered a major hit in 2002 when Mom quit driving, but Jersey's loss was China's gain. Armed with a credit card, a telephone, and a TV tuned to late-night infomercials, her home-shopping phase began. But Michael put a stop to it when he saw all the packages piling up on her front stoop. Losing her ability to buy did not diminish her desire to shop. She constantly hounded others to get her the newest limited-edition Hess truck or the latest McDonald's Happy Meal trinket.

Mom always meant well and occasionally hit a home run. When she ran out of daughters, she started collecting silverware—for me. I joked I was the only straight man with a hope chest. She acquired enough settings for a family of twelve by trading in her Campbell's soup coupons.

Even though I never married, my family of one uses that silverware to this day.

My earliest memory involved both Mom and shopping. At two years old, I tagged along on my first bargain-hunting adventure. Mom's left hand held mine as her right rummaged through the clothing racks at a feverish pace. I did my best to keep up, but it didn't take long for me to get tired and want to stop this shopping thing. My sore back and aching feet along with my hunger to explore the unfamiliar world in my midst took over. A momentary lapse in my mother letting go of my hand presented the perfect opportunity for me to slip free.

After exploring the massive store on my own, I ventured to the great outdoors. There I spotted a pedestrian bridge spanning Route 4's six-lane highway.

That looks like fun, I thought, and I headed straight for it, determined to reach the top.

I climbed up more steps that day than I had so far in my entire life. Maybe not an Olympic feat for most, but it was medal-worthy for a two-year-old. I stopped at the summit to catch my breath and rest my weary legs. The chain-link fence kept me safe as I stood on my tiptoes and peered through. I was mesmerized by the sight and sound of the steady stream of cars racing below.

More stores and more adventures beckoned me from the other side, so I walked across and climbed down what seemed like a million steps. At the bottom, while deciding which way to go, a big blue pickup truck stopped in front of me. A nice-looking man rolled down his window.

"Are you lost?" he asked.

I shrugged. "Guess so."

Another first: a ride in a truck. And then another: he took me to a bar, sat me on the counter, and offered me a Coke on the rocks.

This just might be the best day of my life.

The local barflies, intrigued by my presence, approached. While I enjoyed my drink and made new friends, the man in the truck—an off-duty policeman—got on the phone. Soon after, my mom rushed in, huffing and puffing. How he'd found her I'll never know, but I was glad he did because hanging around in a bar all day had quickly lost its charm.

A morning that began with great promise nearly ended with two-year-old me in a bar, drowning my sorrows with a bunch of drunks. My mom, who willingly—though I'm not sure how willingly—gave up her search for bargains to rescue her youngest child and saved the day. So for me, it was a happy ending. The only loser that day was the Bergen Mall, but I'm sure Mom made up for it on her next uninterrupted trip.

CHAPTER 8

Be Patient

Mom: (distressed) I'm going.
Me: Oh no, is this it?
Mom: (after a moment) I finished.
Me: What?
Mom: Peeing.

After several days of little change, my siblings and I came to terms that our mother was leaving us, comforted only by the fact that she appeared to be in no pain. We took turns sleeping next to her, just in case. Though Mom spoke no words, she responded by squeezing our hands, shifting her body, or moaning softly when we touched foreheads. On the rare occasion when she opened her eyes, she focused solely on the upper corner of the room. Was someone beckoning her? She wouldn't say.

We invited the grandchildren and great-grandchildren to come and say their last goodbyes to their Grandma Zennie. We notified Our Lady of Mount Carmel Catholic Church, where Mom attended Mass for over sixty years. They dispatched a priest who delivered a halfhearted Last Rites. My brother David, who was the only practicing Catholic sibling left, slipped him a tip for his trouble. I was tempted to ask for a refund.

Mom would be buried next to Dad at Valleau Cemetery, a few blocks away. Only one major decision remained: the coffin. On a break, Deecy and I walked to the local funeral home and chose an eco-friendly one. Then we waited. But some waited better than others.

Laurel looked into turning off Mom's pacemaker to quicken the inevitable. "What's the big whoop? If she wants to go, let's help her."

Mom seemed at peace, not suffering in any way. How that thought had ever entered my "born-again" sister's mind, let alone her heart, appalled me. Perhaps "we all grieve in our own way" works here too. Sure, back in 1997, I had dark thoughts about ending my dad's suffering during his final days, but my wish was to end *his* misery, not my own.

Hospice's initial assessment: her body was shutting down. Food was no longer necessary. Ice chips would provide some relief as she transitioned. We obeyed the "no food, ice chips only" directive, and we expected the daily stream of hospice nurses to obey it as well. However, we discovered that nurses often ignored their supervisors and instead dispensed their own brand of care. To make sure they followed the rules, Deecy and I stopped them at the front door with the directive in hand.

This worked well until one nurse glanced at it, approached our mother, and blurted out, "Are you hungry?"

We practically leaped over the bed to shut her up. But, as if hearing a dinner bell, Mom's eyes snapped open. Seeing that, the nurse accused us of starving her to death. She called the office and repeated her accusation. Her supervisor told her to leave, and she did so in a huff.

But now with that thought ringing in my head, I couldn't ignore the possibility. Were we starving our mother to death? Could that rebel nurse be right, and the initial assessment be wrong? Mom showed no signs of hunger or desire for food in weeks, but holy shit, maybe we were.

Racked with guilt, I rushed to her bedside and asked, "Are you hungry, Mom?"

She instantly perked up. "Whaddaya got?" Her first words in weeks.

Shocked, I offered, "Anything you want."

She considered for a moment. "How about some pumpkin pie?"

March was not exactly pumpkin-pie season, but Michael accepted the challenge, and by some small miracle, he returned with not one but two pumpkin pies.

Mom spit out the first spoonful.

That didn't go so well, I thought.

But I tried again to great success. Maybe too great. Totally energized, she downed half a pie. The next day she finished the second pie and then moved on to sherbet, and only sherbet, eight bowls a day. Normally a cause for concern, we ignored the high sugar intake for the time being. Mom was back, and she punctuated her return with a zinger for me.

"I haven't seen you in a *long* while," referring to my long absence.

"I know, Mom. Sorry," was the only response I could muster.

A few days later, when Deecy was alone with her, she asked, "Who was in the corner of the room?"

Mom didn't respond.

"Was it God?"

She shot Deecy a knowing look but remained silent.

Deecy pressed. "Did He speak to you?"

Mom smiled and nodded.

"What did He say?"

"Be patient," she whispered.

CHAPTER 9

The Surviving Catholic

*I sat outside the confessional and timed how long
the girls spent in the box. The longer in,
the more sins they'd committed.
These were the girls I wanted to date. —Me*

Compared to the Cagneys' twelve, the Corcorans' thirteen, or the Cermacs' fourteen, the Porro sixpack barely registered on Our Lady of Mount Carmel's radar; however, the Catholic Church loomed large on ours.

I enrolled in parochial school, as did my older brothers and sisters. I attended Mass on Sundays and Holy Days, and dutifully dropped coins in the collection basket. When I couldn't avoid it, I endured the excruciating ten o'clock High Mass where vocally challenged priests, and I'm being kind here, *sang* a capella so off-key it rattled the stained-glass windows, made the neighborhood dogs howl, and put the fear of God in me for sure.

I ate fish on Fridays, said grace before every meal, and, like Dad, prayed on my knees at night. And every year I gave up candy for Lent for forty endless days. However, by Catholic Law, we could indulge on Sundays. My brothers and I would spring from our beds at the stroke of midnight and gorge ourselves on our sweet hidden treasure until we collapsed in diabetic comas.

To enter the Gates of Heaven, you just had to obey the Ten Commandments. If not, you had to go to church, confess your sins, and say some prayers, and all would be forgiven. While it wasn't much of a deterrent, it was something I relied on more times than I'd ever admit in a court of law. Your first confession was a big deal. You needed to do it before you received your first Holy Communion, which was an even bigger deal.

The morning of my first Holy Communion began in confusion. I'd finished the first grade and considered myself a second grader. Over breakfast, my sister Laurel insisted that I wasn't "officially" a second grader until school started in September. So, when I pulled back that velvet curtain in the confessional, slipped into the pitch-black box, and knelt on that uncomfortable step—I guess to remind me of my unworthiness—I hoped the kind, understanding priest would help settle the debate. My heart raced as I listened to his muffled voice behind the latticed window. I shifted back and forth on my aching knees, waiting and waiting. When the muttering stopped, I was overcome with a sudden and intense urge to pee, which made me want to escape. But as the window slid open, I froze.

An imposing shadow spoke in a calm voice. "You may begin."

Thawing quickly, I stammered through my not-so-well-rehearsed lines. "Um, bless me, um, Father."

"Go on," the shadow said.

Silence.

The shadow prompted, "For I have sinned..." *You too?* I didn't say that, but wished I had. Instead, my tongue remained tied.

Then the shadow's calm tone turned sharp. "How old are you?"

I perked up. "Okay, so I think I'm in the second grade, but my sister says I'm not."

"Come back when you're old enough."

I'm six, give me a break. But before I could finish that thought, the window slammed shut, and along with it went my hopes of being absolved from my sins, my trust in priests, and my faith in the whole idea of confession. And besides, my knees were hurting and I had to pee.

My first confession wasn't the only traumatic incident I experienced at Mount Carmel. When filling in for a sick altar boy—with no official training other than the Meyer brothers' last-minute instructions—I stumbled more than once. Father Patrick ripped into me sotto voce throughout the service and then for everyone to hear by the end. Thus ended any notion I had of becoming an altar boy.

As far as I knew, the priests at Mount Carmel "behaved." The ones I remember—Father Quinn, Father Finn, and Monsignor Kelly—were ancient, much older than my dad. It seemed like you had to be Irish in order to be a priest in our church. The Monsignor also sat on the police board. Two years later, his power and influence saved me after a flash of juvenile delinquency got the best of me. Thankful, I raced to confession after that, but I made sure to pee beforehand.

The nuns came right out of Disney central casting, black habits and all. Sister Josephina, our principal, wielded her power fairly. Sister Margaret Jones, my first nun crush, was young, and as far as I could tell, pretty. My second crush was Sister Ann from the film *The Singing Nun*. Mount Carmel's Sister Rita and her aquiline nose both had character. The strict, unforgiving, square-jawed Sister Laura took pride in playing judge and jury and delivering swift verdicts and harsh punishment.

One day, a student got hurt on the asphalt playground during morning recess. *Who thought monkey bars on asphalt was a good idea?* At afternoon recess, I apparently crossed Sister Laura's unknown, invisible, and forbidden line safeguarding the spot where it happened.

Faux tough-guy Ken turned me in. (Ken would reappear three years later to cause me even more trouble.) He hauled me into Sister Laura's court, and before I uttered a word, she rendered her verdict: guilty.

With no ruler to rap my knuckles, she slapped me across the face and asked, "How does that feel?"

It was a light touch compared to what my older brothers doled out, so I stifled a smile and said nothing. In hindsight, I wish I had the presence of mind to turn the other cheek just to freak her out.

That slap was the last straw for my parents. The following year, David and I enrolled at Travell Elementary. But the transition from parochial to public school wasn't as smooth as I'd hoped.

Early in the year, my fourth-grade class teamed up with another for game day. My opponent cheated. When I called her out, she denied it. So I slapped her, just like Sister Laura slapped me, and said, "Cheating is a sin."

She burst into tears.

Then my teacher, Mrs. Hopkins, made a beeline for us. My adrenaline spiked. The terrifying thought of going back to Mount Carmel flashed before my eyes. For the life of me, I can't recall what I said or did, but I became that girl's best friend in a matter of seconds. By the time Mrs. Hopkins arrived at our desk, the two of us were all smiles. She eyed us suspiciously for what seemed like an eternity before moving on. Even though I never struck a girl or a woman again, I learned the power and mystery of "charm" that day. It was a valuable lesson that I would benefit from throughout my life. In fact, I won the "Best at Charming Themselves Out of Trouble" trophy in the seventh grade, and I didn't even know that award existed.

The Catholic students who were attending public school continued our religious training in Catechism classes on Tuesday nights. These casual affairs were held in the teacher's home and were social events more than anything else. By the ninth grade, I became disenchanted with the whole "church" thing. I had too many questions. When I began asking them, the teachers branded me an atheist.

"One does not question what's written in the Bible," they would say.

Well, *this* one did. Even though we had a Catholic Bible in our house, I don't recall anyone ever reading it, including my dad, who attended Mass every day at 6:30 a.m. since he was thirteen years old. Maybe he got his fill there. Our family Bible was where Mom recorded important family events in her elegant handwriting—births, with dates and times, First Holy Communions and Confirmations, childhood diseases, injuries, surgeries, marriages, and one divorce. I never questioned what Mom wrote in the Bible.

When I voiced my concerns with the Church to my father, he suggested I speak with a priest. When the priest offered no good answers, I stopped attending Mass. What saved me from my devout dad's wrath was my declaration beforehand: "I can no longer go to a church that can't answer fair questions."

Dad took my hiatus from church in stride, or so I thought. A few days later, he handed me a typewritten letter. In it, he defended the Church and justified his duty as a Catholic father. I saved his heartfelt letter for decades and only recently can't remember where I put it for safekeeping—apparently in an excellent hiding place.

After a brief return while in college, I abandoned the Catholic Church for good, but not all its teachings. Over time, I grew to appreciate them more and more. I learned the difference between right and wrong, to put others before yourself, and to honor thy father and mother. And despite my first confession trauma and Sister Laura's slap, I do have many fond memories of my time at Our Lady of Mount Carmel.

My mornings began with Pillsbury cinnamon rolls. The thought of them still makes my mouth water. David and I inventing games while waiting for the school bus was always fun. The five who attended Our Lady of Mount Carmel were left-handed, yet no one made any attempt to change us. This was quite unusual since many in the Church declared lefties as Servants of the Devil.

Whenever people asked my right-handed parents, "Where did all those southpaws come from?" I would joke, "Our mailman was a lefty."

My issues with the Catholic dogma in no way swayed my opinion regarding the excellent, well-rounded education I received in my four years. Not only did they teach the basics— reading, writing, and arithmetic—but they also taught us about the arts and art history. From weaving my first potholder, to drawing my first and only cross-eyed Santa with movable arms and legs, to painting my first still life, to studying classic paintings that I would one day stand in front of in New York and Paris, my interest in the arts has never waned.

CHAPTER 10

It Took a Theft

Swear to God, I saw her heart break. —Me

Why we started remains uncertain, but how we started was crystal clear. Like many addictions, it all started with just one, but one cigarette was not enough. One became two, two became three, three became four, five, six. Soon, packs of twenty weren't enough. As the curse of addiction sank its claws deeper and deeper, we jonesed for more and more. Packs became cartons, then multiple cartons, and when those failed to satisfy, we spiced it up with cigars and Tiparillos with the plastic tips. Still, enough was never enough.

Me and the Meyer twins called ourselves the Cigarette Bandits. We didn't wear masks, just innocent faces. We were ten years old, and we were good at this game. We weren't addicted to smoking—that's not what drove us. It was the heart-pounding thrill of stealing that drove us. We could have stolen candy, snacks, anything else, but we chose cigarettes for some reason. Maybe we wanted to be like our television and movie heroes. Maybe we figured no one in our town would suspect young boys of shoplifting cartons of cigarettes on a sunny summer afternoon. Or maybe going full rebel as Catholics meant smoking or drinking, but bottles made too much noise and were too heavy for our getaway bikes. So, cigarettes it was, and then cigars and Tiparillos.

Our prime target was the Grand Union. It was located downtown and close to our hideout. It offered a diverse tobacco section and several escape routes. The local A&P had fewer options, but it was our backup. Our plan was simple. Our execution, flawless. We parked our bikes around the corner and out of sight. We brought our own brown paper bag that matched the store's brand. Two stood as lookouts at opposite ends of the cigarette aisle while the third stuffed the bag with full cartons. We left the bag and roamed the store to make sure we didn't attract suspicion. If we did, we would slip away and try our luck at the A&P. If the coast was clear, we grabbed the bag, waltzed our way out, jumped on our bikes, and rode like the wind to freedom.

Freedom was a loft in an abandoned garage near the twins' house. After each haul, we divvied up the loot and celebrated by firing up a cigar, cigarette, or Tiparillo. We didn't smoke, not really, only pretended to. Still, we had our favorites. Newport menthols were mine. The twins favored Benson & Hedges 100s. No one liked Marlboros or filter-less Camels because they were too strong. But that didn't stop us from adding them to the kitty along with Kents, Pall Malls, Winstons, and Lucky Strikes.

We never got caught red-handed, only red-faced, when the owner of the garage walked in on us after a major haul. He took one look at the packs of cigarettes and said, "Damn, and I just quit smoking last month."

He let us walk away scot-free if we left the loot. The Cigarette Bandits disbanded soon after.

I could blame the television series *It Takes a Thief*, or movies like Hitchcock's *To Catch a Thief*, for making crime so damn attractive, or the influence of my questionable friends, or my competitive spirit. But the truth is, I liked the rush.

Two years later, that rush would lead me to the worst day of my young life. I became quite proficient at picking bicycle locks. After Sunday school, I'd head out to the bike racks to test my skills. I'd open and close them, then move to the next. No harm done. Faux tough-guy Ken— yes, that Ken, Sister Laura's lackey—and his friend were also trying to pick locks, but with less success.

"Hey, that's a nice one. Why not take it?" Ken said when he saw me free a brand-new Stingray bike.

I didn't need the bike or want it, but I took it anyway. Peer pressure? Perhaps. Just to play it safe, I stashed the bike in a friend's garage and headed home.

As I cut through a neighbor's yard, I spotted a police car parked in front of my house. It appeared Ken had turned me in yet again. Safe to say, I could have used less of Ken in my life. My heart pounded. My gut twisted into knots. This was not the kind of rush I was looking for, and there was no way I was going home until the police left. I hid in the bushes and prepared my defense.

As the police taillights faded down Emmett Place, I took a few deep breaths, mustered up my innocence, and entered the side door. Mom greeted me and wasted no time.

"Did you steal a bicycle today?"

I looked her straight in the eye and said, "No."

She seemed relieved. "Okay."

She had no reason to think I was lying but taking no chances I escaped to the safety of my bedroom.

Did I just get away with it? And if so, for how long?

Not long, it turned out. Racked with guilt, I returned to the kitchen within minutes and confessed. Mom handled it with grace, but in that moment, I swear to God I saw her heart break.

She confirmed it when she said, "Your lie hurt more than your stealing the bike."

I never lied to her again.

CHAPTER 11

Planting the Seed

Mom: I don't like you swearing.
Me: I'm sorry. It's tough being a parent.
Mom: I guess. But I never swore.

Well-schooled by hospice, Deecy and I became proficient in tending to our mother's daily needs, including sponge baths, bedsore treatment, diaper, clothes, and bedding changes—not easy with the helpless patient lying in bed.

Seeing Mom naked the first time, though uncomfortable, was something I had to get over quickly. There was work to do. However, seeing what aging had done to her body took a bit more effort. Scars from her 1998 triple bypass surgery were prominent. Her once-full breasts resembled low-hanging saddle bags. Above the left one, a pacemaker the size of a bottle cap protruded from under her skin. She had very little body hair, which I regarded as a plus and something to look forward to as I was already tired of shaving my ears.

During our stay, we took over most duties, taking breaks only when hospice paid their daily visits. Mom was now sitting up, alert, smiling, talking, eating umpteen bowls of sherbet, and only sherbet. The flavor didn't matter—lemon, lime, watermelon, raspberry— just keep it coming. Her if-you-don't-already-have-diabetes-you-will-surely-get-it-now diet lasted for several weeks. Sherbet might not have been the smartest medicine, but that's all she wanted. And who were we to question this eighty-nine-year-old phoenix who rose from the dead with renewed youth and energy? Genevieve was back and in the pink.

With Mom on the mend, Deecy headed home to East Grand Rapids, but not without her ever-present second thoughts. Her type A personality caused her to question everything, especially her own decisions, and this was a big one. Should she stay or should she go? As the airport limo pulled away from the house, the Middle Eastern driver noticed her sobbing in the back seat and asked why. Her tearful explanation ignited his passionate response:

"There is no more important thing for a child to do than to take care of their parents in their twilight years. I left my home and my family to care for my ailing father for two long years. It nearly cost me my job, my marriage, and my own family, but I regret nothing."

His story sent Deecy reeling, bringing even more tears. Her sacrifice had only been three weeks, but she needed to return to her job, her husband, and her five children. Torn and tempted to have the driver turn back until another set of second thoughts intervened. She continued on to Michigan.

When Deecy shared the driver's story, it struck an emotional chord in me. I could be selfish. As the fifth-born child of six, it was easy to be. I fought for attention and respect. Sometimes I fought just for the sake of fighting. I didn't do anything I didn't want to. If I wanted something, I took it. My sister-in-law recently reminded me of my brother David's forty-year grudge regarding this. On steak night, as a healthy slab of overcooked beef made its way around the dinner table, we each cut our own piece and passed the plate. When my turn came, if the best piece—closest to the bone—was there for the taking, it was mine. I never gave it a second thought.

However, one Christmas things began to change for me. Per Michael's suggestion, the Porro kids broke from tradition. We bought one hundred oranges and spent a good part of our Christmas Day passing them out at local nursing homes. The seniors, who had no other visitors that day, welcomed us like we were the Three Kings and treated our oranges like they were gold, frankincense, and myrrh. As an eleven-year-old, I wasn't too keen on this idea at first, but that experience had a profound effect on me. I can still see the smiles on their faces and the joy in their eyes as we handed them oranges and said, "Merry Christmas."

Since then, I'd found my sweet spot as a giver.

At fifteen, I experienced my favorite Christmas of all time. I gave my parents the award-winning coffee table, and I carved a unique cherrywood statue for each of my siblings and my two brothers-in-law. Their heart-warming responses moved me to tears and forever cemented my role.

I gave away all the furniture pieces I crafted in high school: my buffet to Caryl, my china cabinet to Laurel, and my Governor Winthrop desk landed in its rightful place in Deecy's home. I created one-of-a-kind greeting cards for my family. These came to be expected and sorely missed when I got distracted, which happened often while I was away at college. During one of my mother's visits, she noticed several handmade cards sitting on my girlfriend's desk.

"I guess this is why we don't see these too much anymore," Mom said.

Guilt trip noted. You can bet she got a special handmade card that Mother's Day. Those cards and their trademarked character, Mr. Nobody, inspired the first of my unintentional nonprofit business adventures: The Marcard Greeting Card Company.

I wrote poems recapping highlights of our annual family reunions. In 1995, I filmed *Ciao Celle*, a documentary of Dad's and my trip to Italy so everyone could discover what we discovered. For monumental birthdays, I designed unique books and boxes filled with photographs and memories. The first were solo efforts for Dad and Mom, then I asked family and friends to contribute to the ones for my siblings and my aunts. I also gave them as wedding gifts to my nieces and nephews. The unveiling became a popular event as all gathered around to see what Uncle Mark had created this time.

To be clear, I didn't totally give up being selfish, as I consider all this giving to be somewhat self-serving. The expectation, the reactions, and the appreciation pleased me to no end.

I might not have realized it at the time, but Deecy's limo driver, like the Christmas oranges, planted a seed in me.

CHAPTER 12

A Recurring Dream

*A major function of dreams is the
fulfillment of wishes.*
—Sigmund Freud

T hroughout my childhood, I experienced a few recurring dreams: falling from great heights or caught in a suffocating riptide, always waking up in the nick of time. Those dreams didn't stop me from climbing trees and rooftops, or swimming in the ocean, and they eventually went away. But the one I dreamed about the most did not and remained a bit of a mystery.

It's in black-and-white. I am five or six years old. Mom and I are alone in a rowboat gliding across a foggy, gray, eerily quiet lake. I'm sitting up front, peering over the bow on the lookout for logs, debris, or rocks that might impede us.

Mom, young, beautiful with long wavy hair—no doubt inspired by old photos—sits at the stern. In command, with oars in hand, she rows with a purpose, but it was anybody's guess as to where we were headed. As they say in boating, "It's not about the destination, it's about the journey." She rows facing me, which I found odd, but in a child's dream, mothers can do the impossible. We speak no words, and though the setting appears gloomy, neither of us seems particularly concerned.

Freud would have a field day with this dream and would probably find all kinds of Oedipus-complex themes in it. But I'd like to think it's simply about a mother guiding her young son through the murky waters of childhood. With an often-disappointed father, two older sisters who repeatedly tried to tickle me to death, and two overzealous brothers who attempted the same fate by other methods, life for me—an overly sensitive, bedwetting, thumb-sucking asthmatic—did indeed get murky. However, the boat in the dream is my safe place, and all is calm within it. I trusted Mom to navigate around all obstacles that lay ahead.

All these years later, I can reinterpret that dream to reflect our current journey. Instead of a mother guiding her son, it was the reverse. I was the captain, out front, identifying—and now removing—all obstacles impeding us. The boat remained our safe place. Neither Mom nor I seemed concerned because I was in command. Remember, it's not about the destination. Mom had put her trust in me. I may be guiding the way, but she, with oars in hand, controlled when and how this journey ended.

This was not our first jaunt through life's murky waters. We were together when she had a small stroke in 1972, a major stroke in 1993, a triple bypass surgery in 1998, and a trip to the emergency room on the night of my twenty-fifth high school reunion in 2000. And now we once again found ourselves in the same boat. Freud said that a major function of dreams is the fulfillment of wishes. Was this our destiny? Was this my wish fulfilled?

CHAPTER 13

Salt, Pepper, and a Dash of Whiskey

Mom: Why are you so good to me?
Me: Because you're my mom and I love you.
Mom: You're a good kid.
Me: (under my breath) The meds are working.

My brother Michael, six years my senior, was the first to witness our mother's unconditional love for even the tiniest member of our family. In the early 1960s, we had plenty of cats, six by my count. So, when Mom brought home two baby mice—one white and one black—it was perfectly reasonable to wonder why. After all, this was enemy territory, and Salt and Pepper were nothing but easy, yet tasty, prey. However, our cats were well-behaved, and they welcomed the fresh additions with open paws, as did Michael. And so began his love affair with these furry little creatures.

He could often be found with his nose pressed against the glass of Salt and Pepper's cage, locking eyes with them. They seemed as curious about Michael as he was about them. Both mice were sociable but had distinct personalities, with Salt being the more affectionate of the two. They were neat, clean, and constantly groomed themselves, industrious too. They created comfy wonders with tissues and toilet paper rolls. Both loved to exercise, either by going nowhere on their mouse-propelled wheel or on the endless trek running from Michael's one hand to the other. But because they were delicate, he learned to handle them with care.

Michael didn't know what gender Salt or Pepper were, but after a few weeks the mating chase began and left no doubt. They raced around the cage until Salt finally surrendered to Pepper's charms. After a few more weeks, Michael witnessed the miracle of birth. He watched in awe as Salt, in full control, licked each pup clean, and made sure each took their first breath before the next arrived, and the next, and so on. Pepper played his part as the doting father, even though these pups looked nothing like mice: bald, translucent, eyes and ears closed. However, it didn't take long—just days—for them to open their eyes and don their familiar fur coats. It also didn't take long for a new chase to begin. Salt and Pepper became breeding machines, producing many mouse pups several times a year, which gave birth to a new and profitable business for Michael, selling mice to the Ye Towne Pet Shop for ten cents apiece. Big money back then.

The lifespan of mice is short, maybe two years. So, sadly, Salt and Pepper also taught Michael about death. After many litters, Salt slowed down until one night she appeared ready to call it quits. Michael resigned himself to the inevitable, but not Mom. She made several attempts to revive Salt. First with cheese, then with water, but to no avail. She heated a hot water bottle and lay Salt on it. Still no change. But Mom didn't give up. Michael drifted in and out of sleep while she stayed awake, determined to nurse that little mouse back to health.

Finally, in the wee hours and out of options, Mom resorted to an old wives' tale. She dashed off to the kitchen and returned with a bottle of whiskey. In itself, a miracle. Liquor was present in our house for one reason and one reason only: Mom's Christmas Whiskey Balls. A blurry-eyed Michael watched Mom fill an eyedropper with the "water of life" and place a drop on Salt's lips. That mouse perked right up, got back on her feet, and moved about like her young self. An old wives' tale? As Dad would say, "Bunk." But it worked. Salt went on to live many more mouse years and produced many more pups, which earned Michael many more dimes.

Mom's devotion to animals shouldn't have come as a surprise. We witnessed it many times over the years. She always jumped in to give our pets the love and attention they deserved whenever ours waned. And she always took good care of them until the bitter end. But on that night, a young boy saw it for the first time and learned an indelible lesson.

And even though that old wives' tale played a role in plenty more pet revivals, Michael knew it was his mother's love—more than the whiskey—that brought each of them back.

CHAPTER 14

My "I'm from Missour-uh" Mom and My Brother Teresa

Me: Where do you find these people?

Michael: God sends them to me.

W hen Mom doubted my tall tales, she declared, "I'm from Missour-uh." I never understood that as a child. As a born-and-bred "New Yawker," why in the world would she claim she was from anywhere else? And where did the "uh" come from? It's spelled Missouri, with an *i*, that's pronounced, *ee*, which also made no sense and only amplified my confusion.

Dad's "Son of a gun" or "Ya bagrat" clearly captured the Brooklyn brashness we all knew and loved. Did Mom secretly prefer the mighty Mississippi over the Hudson River? *Show Boat* over *Guys and Dolls*? The Cardinals over the Yankees? Apparently, yes. Her favorite musical featured her favorite song, "Why Do I Love You?" Her upright piano music box chimed the same tune. She even named her Bichon Frisé, Zuri, as in, "I'm from . . ."

It's widely accepted that in 1899, Representative Willard D. Vandiver coined the famous phrase, "Frothy eloquence neither convinces nor satisfies me. I'm from Missouri. You've got to show me," and Missourians latched on to it ever since.

My frothy eloquence got me out of plenty of trouble over the years, but never with Mom. Whenever she said, "I'm from Missour-uh," I heard, "I don't believe you," and I knew I was in trouble. That phrase caused me a lot of grief in the past, and it caused those who were less than sincere a lot of grief in the present. Which brings us to Tammy and the Tweedles.

My brother Michael's penchant for rescuing sick animals in his youth evolved into hiring the wrong people for the right reasons as an adult. He'd give any needy person a chance, or two, or three. Unfortunately, most didn't deserve his gift or appreciate his charitable nature. Which again brings us to Tammy and the Tweedles.

Three years ago, Michael interviewed and hired Tweedle Dee. Shortly after, she arrived with her toddler; her mother, Tweedle Dumb; a pitifully overweight dog, a bird, a goldfish, and a black cat. And they wasted no time making our house their home.

It couldn't have been easy for Mom. She must have felt like a prisoner. She had some say in the matter, but other than "I do not want to return to assisted living," she kept quiet—at least with us. So, with limited options, we accepted less than ideal. As it turned out, far less.

In the beginning, the Tweedles seemed like a lovely family. They got along well with Mom, and she with them. However, their contempt for her cropped up early. Although they hid it well from Michael, they must have shown their true nature to our "I'm from Missour-uh" mother, and tensions mounted. Yet the Tweedles stayed put and kept quiet—at least with us.

Michael suspected these three generations escaped from a desperate situation in upstate New York, so he took pity on them. He brushed aside the early warning signs and instead cut the Tweedles break after break. And they embraced each and every one. They had a sweet deal, and they made it even sweeter by doing less and less of what we hired them to do and more and more of what they wanted.

I noticed hints during my visits. The echoes of past friction lingered in this house. They sat Mom facing the kitchen wall for all her meals while they muttered behind her back. When she fell asleep watching Animal Planet, Tweedle Dumb snuck in and turned it off, ignoring the fact that there's no quicker way to wake someone from a deep sleep than to turn off the TV. And whenever Tweedle Dee, who expressed herself best through baking, surprised Mom, a type 2 diabetic, with a super sweet treat, one that would catapult even a non-diabetic into sugar shock, I questioned her motives.

Maybe I was overly sensitive to it, maybe not. I've got a little of my Mom's "I'm from Missour-uh" in me too. The Tweedles' fake smiles couldn't make the sad meals they served taste better, or make the messy house look cleaner. Their syrupy baby talk couldn't hide the fact that Mom just did not look happy with them around.

"She's not a child," I said to Tweedle Dumb. "Why do you talk to her like that?"

She giggled. "She loves it when I call her 'Jennie Bennie.'"

Mom's expression said otherwise.

My siblings also sensed the tension, but those of us who lived far away had it easy. We swooped in, complained to Michael, and swooped back out. None of us were willing or able to take on his responsibilities. It must have weighed on him, but the thought of interviewing, hiring, and onboarding yet another team was unbearable. So, he bit his tongue and kept lowering the bar of expectation so as to not disturb the ever-plunging status quo. And we continued to yield to his credo. "Having warm bodies in the house in case of an emergency was better than nothing."

Not by much, it turns out. Last summer, Mom fell on her way to the bathroom and gashed her forehead. Tweedle Dee and Tweedle Dumb's warm bodies were of little help. These two plus-sized women dared not attempt to get Mom up and to the hospital or call 911. Instead, they trudged to our next-door neighbor, who weighed 135 pounds and was recovering from a recent heart attack and begged him to come to the rescue. Thankfully, he did. And fortunately, both survived, but Mom's injury required a lengthy hospital stay. That should have been the tipping point.

I didn't hear about Mom's fall until long after the incident. Like I said, those of us who lived far away had it easy, especially if we were kept in the dark. Did my being too sensitive cause the silence? Perhaps. When I finally heard the full story, and then read my brother David's thank-you note to the Tweedles—which they proudly displayed on the refrigerator—I almost gagged.

Michael kept the Tweedles on, but after Mom returned from the hospital, he hired Tammy, a forty-something, self-proclaimed nurse's aide who desperately needed a job. This was music to my Brother Teresa's ears. But her lack of skill and training became crystal clear when hospice arrived to assess their new patient, the environment, and to remove any hazards.

Janice, the no-nonsense lead nurse, entered a bedroom where a nearly combustible stench of urine hung in the air. Amid the fog, she discovered my unresponsive mother with infected bedsores so deep you could lose your finger in them.

"This patient has not been properly cared for," Janice declared, then demanded, "Who's responsible?" With the spotlight laser-focused on Tammy, she braced for a fight. Fireworks erupted when Janice determined the only hazard was Tammy. That, too, should have been the tipping point.

First impressions are like scars, impossible to erase. When I first saw Tammy slumped in the corner, resisting Janice's training, I feared the worst. I sensed that tough chick hardened by a rough life on the wrong side of town was a ticking time bomb and if crossed, *boom!*

Although I've experienced my share of blind spots, I tend to read most people quickly and accurately. Years of acting training and studying human behavior sharpened that skill. If I feel you don't deserve a break, you might get one, but you won't get another. Michael practiced the opposite, no matter how many red flags waved.

To be fair, when Mom moved back to 247, Michael stepped up big time. He handled her finances, ran errands, scheduled doctor's appointments, administered medications, hired the help, and checked in often. His efforts provided great comfort to us, and having warm bodies, any warm bodies in the house when his wasn't, provided great comfort to him.

I love my Brother Teresa, and I applaud his benevolence. I only wish he had more of our mother's "I'm from Missour-uh" in him, and I pray that at least a few of the needy souls God continues to send his way prove worthy of his gifts. Tammy and the Tweedles did not.

CHAPTER 15

The Miracle Poop

Mom: I don't need to go on the commode.

*Me: But you go every night, and I need
to clean you.
Don't you want to be fresh
as a daisy and smell like a rose?
You'll be a bouquet of loveliness.*

(She shoots me a look.)

Mom's nothing-but-sherbet diet gave way to her nothing-but-oatmeal diet—bowls and bowls of sugary-sweet oatmeal. We kept her hydrated with an endless supply of Gatorade in their endless variety of fluorescent flavors. We were fully aware she might just be riding the most amazing and continuous sugar high, but to play it safe, we didn't change a thing.

The phrase "no shit" can mean several things. Context and inflection determine which one it is. It could be a question as in, "Are you telling me the truth?" A wisecrack after someone stated the obvious, as in, "No shit, Sherlock." Or a demand as in, "Don't lie to me." However, if you literally mean "no shit," as in one hasn't, that's a problem, one that could lead to serious health issues.

With Mom stuck in bed but eating regularly, *that* issue reared its ugly head, or in her case, had yet to. She peed often—evidenced by the number of diapers we changed each day—but she hadn't pooped in weeks. If her bowels didn't move, her body couldn't eliminate wastes and toxins, and life-threatening complications could result. So, one way or another, that poop had to come out.

Mom being bedridden only complicated things. Janice, the lead hospice nurse, proposed extraction, then donned a latex glove. I then realized what I was in for. Having had some experience with this sort of thing helped me proceed, though not without trepidation.

My annual medical checkups always included a Digital Rectal Exam in which my doctor's semi-familiar finger probed my inner sanctum to detect prostate problems. To lighten the mood, I always asked him to dim the lights, put on some jazz music, then added a friendly warning. "If I turn around and see you smiling, I'll kick your ass."

Undaunted, he slipped on a glove—punctuated with a *snap*—dipped his digit in K-Y jelly, and commanded, "Drop 'em and bend over." Although necessary, it was not my favorite procedure.

It was shocking enough when I saw Mom naked for the first time a mere few weeks ago. I think I handled that okay. Though awkward, it was necessary to get over it and get on with it. But what I was about to do would redefine our relationship *forever*. I took a deep breath, grabbed a latex glove, and slipped it on.

While Mom lay on her side, Janice and I took turns extracting what we could with our gloved fingers. Mom's entire body shuddered with every attempt. Mine did too. It's debatable who got the shorter end of *that* stick, but being a good son, I'll say Mom.

This procedure proved to be not only uncomfortable for all participants, but in the end, unsuccessful. Janice then suggested letting gravity do its thing. However, getting Mom up and into the bathroom through the narrow doorway in her fragile condition was too risky. Then I remembered we had bought Dad a bedside commode fourteen years ago, one that held a special memory.

Two days before he passed, I lifted him and his two hundred pounds of deadweight off that commode. Mom stood by at the ready with a roll of toilet paper. Dad, wishing to hold on to one of his few remaining dignities, insisted on wiping himself. He asked for two sheets.

"Just two sheets?" Mom countered.

"I'm very accurate," he replied.

We all burst out laughing, and I nearly dropped him. I relish that moment. It was one of the last laughs we shared, and it continues to tickle me to this day.

Knowing our family's recycling history, there was a good chance that commode was still in this house.

Our introduction to recycling came early. If food scraps didn't make it into Dad's kitchen creations, they ended up in the compost pile next to the garage. Now, decades later, that soil might be the most fertile in the entire Garden State. But my father's passion for recycling extended far beyond food.

He turned pie tins into lamp shades, shoelaces into lamp cords, and brown paper bags into schoolbook covers. Gift wrapping that wasn't torn to shreds was used to wrap gifts again and again. Even our old refrigerator door found a new life. After years of steady service, our Frigidaire had finally conked out and a new one soon replaced it. Having no further use, hauling fridge to the curb on junk day would have been a fitting farewell, unless you were my dad. He said goodbye only to the cabinet. The fridge door had a new purpose, a reincarnation. Once stripped of its chrome handle, shelves, and insulation, and after adding a rope handle to hold on to for dear life, that door did what no flexible flyer or toboggan could on a fresh fallen blanket of snow. It provided a pilot and six willing passengers thirty thrilling seconds of barely controllable fun sliding down Maryann Place, a short, steep, and—as long as friends stopped traffic at the bottom—safe hill, much to the envy of all onlookers, many of whom lined up for their turn.

Things that left our house, whether obsolete, broken, or even dangerous, rarely left for long. If there was any chance of a new life, Dad stuffed it in the rafters above his workshop, in the crawl space behind the laundry chute, or in the garage that in my lifetime never housed a car. I guess you could say there was a method to his madness. The normal cycle went like this: when something no longer served its intended purpose, Dad moved it to the basement. If Mom or one of us kids found it first, we'd put it in the trash or out on the curb for junk day. Upon returning from work, Dad would rescue and hide it in the garage until that day came for repurposing.

It's fair to attribute my father's waste-not-want-not passion to surviving the Great Depression. Mom also grew up during the Depression era and, like Dad, seldom threw anything out. But unlike my father, that never stopped her from buying new things. Mom redecorated rather than repurposed. She refreshed drab furniture with a coat of paint in the hip color of the day. She revitalized old lamps with gold leaf and a new shade. No pie-tin lamp shades or shoelace lamp cords would do for her. And she topped tables, no matter the size or shape, with a custom slab of marble. The only things she repurposed were vacant bedrooms to store all her bargains.

Now, fingers crossed, I headed for the basement in search of the commode. I risked life and limb tiptoeing across the minefield of junk, dead mice, and disturbing memories. There it sat, under the ballet barre where my sisters practiced their pliés and from where David gagged, hogtied, and suspended me until Dad came to my rescue. The commode was plenty dusty but intact.

After a rigorous cleaning, I set it up next to Mom's bed and explained our mission to her. She was more than game since it involved no more poking or prodding.

I barely got the diaper off and her onto the commode before the bucket shook with a heavy thud, taking with it much of the stress and strain on her face. It simply melted away. Her pale complexion faded as rosy cheeks emerged.

Eureka!

Did I dare look in the bucket? I did. My eyes teared. My nostrils flared. My body froze in awe. Two words came to mind. Just two, but they were perfect: "No shit!"

When my nephew Abe's son, Julien, first learned about number one and number two, he emerged from the bathroom after his first solo potty trip and boasted, "Dad, I did a seven."

Well, on the Julien scale, Mom did a *fifty*. She gave birth to one colossal, yet glorious, life-saving piece of shit. How something that humongous came out of her tiny butt while causing no apparent pain was nothing short of a miracle. I held my breath, shot a photo of that wondrous thing, and emailed it to all of my siblings. Reactions ranged from bravo to revulsion, which left no doubt I had found my Christmas card idea. Even decorated with a red bow, I'm sure that image brought the same reactions from the same siblings. Hey, every miracle, big or small, real or imagined, must be celebrated.

I am immensely thankful for two things that night. My parents—the original recyclers who threw nothing out—and to Sir Isaac Newton for discovering gravity. Without them both, that Miracle Poop would not have happened.

CHAPTER 16

Is That Your Picasso in the Outfield?

If I'd only stuck a mitt on my head,
I could have been a Major Leaguer. —Me

Springtime brought the birds, the bees, flowers, green grass, and the start of baseball season, which was a big deal in our house when I was a kid. Dad was a Pony League coach, my two older brothers played, and I *attempted* to play. While America's pastime bonded most fathers and sons, it drove a wedge between Dad and me.

Tiny Tim Baseball presented several challenges for me: focus, or more precisely, maintaining it. I liked baseball, but I also liked art. Playing right field allowed me the opportunity to satisfy both. I was one of the few left-handers in the league. The right-handers rarely hit to the opposite field. Except for a misplayed pop fly or the occasional grounder slipping through the infield gap, I had a lot of free time out there, so I drew pictures in the dirt. If someone yelled, "Hey, Mark, incoming!" I'd chase down the ball, throw it back, and return to my canvas. By the end of the game, I'd collected a hit or two and created an impressive work of art.

But this was not the dual threat my father envisioned for his youngest son. Witnessing this once was enough. He avoided the rest of my games that season and thereby avoided fielding the question, "Is that *your* Picasso in the outfield?"

Dad continued to take time out from his own team to drill into me the fundamentals of baseball, and I continued to show little interest in learning them. Ground balls scared me. Touching your glove to the turf just meant putting your face closer to danger. Catching line drives sent shock waves up my arm. And pop flies? I'll make my issue with them very clear, very soon.

The only thing I looked forward to at practice was when it ended. But one day my interest sparked after we, really just Michael and David, finished infield drills. Dad stood at the plate and launched fly balls deep into the outfield. These were no can-of-corn pop flies; they were Mickey Mantle home runs. I stood in awe as each ball rose skyward and momentarily disappeared beyond the clouds before returning to earth and into my brothers' gloves. Now this looked like my kind of fun.

I grabbed my glove and hustled to the outfield. After watching my brothers shag a few more and make it look easy, I waved my arms, beckoning my dad to send one my way. He all but ignored me. I waved harder and harder until he finally gave in and pointed my way. I bounced in anticipation.

"Okay, here it comes, my very own Mickey Mantle home run." He tossed up the ball and swung his bat.

Crack.

It sounded like a cannon. The ball climbed up and up and up, high into the sky. I stood there, as I saw my brothers had done, and waited and waited. Looking up at that tiny, seemingly harmless white dot, I started thinking.

That ball is really, really high. When it comes down, it will be going really, really fast.

My heart raced. My feet froze.

And it's really going to hurt.

I didn't want any part of that pain, so I broke free and ran to the right. I only got a few steps before that fly ball found my head and knocked me to the ground.

My dad and my brothers traded looks. *Did that just happen?*

As I writhed in pain, all three rushed to my aid. Nothing major, just a lump and a bruised ego. Hoping to temper the inevitable teasing, I dried my tears, got back on my feet, and dusted myself off as Dad trotted back to home plate. *Did he do that on purpose?*

My brothers caught several more balls before I got my nerve up and called for another. Dad resisted, but I flapped my arms like a crazed bird until he caved.

Crack.

Up, up it climbed, higher than the last. But throb, throb went my head.

No way. I'm outta here.

This time I escaped to the left and down I went—again. Two for two. They couldn't believe their eyes. I couldn't believe my head. The pain.

While they wondered if I was gifted in a strange sort of way, I wondered, *Does my father hate me?*

Under normal circumstances, practice should have ended then and there, but "normal" vanished two Mickey-Mantle-home-run fly balls ago. Once again, I struggled to my feet, wiped my tears, and dusted myself off. Blame my bruised and battered ego. Blame the two possible concussions. Or blame my hell-bent need to blunt Michael and David's sure-to-come psychological torture. Whatever the reason, I was determined to prove the first two balls were flukes. I begged for another shot, set myself, and waited.

The crack of his bat sent shivers down my spine. My head throbbed, in stereo.

What the heck was I thinking?

I didn't dare look up. My feet froze again, but this time I took it as a sign and stayed put. I buried my head in my chest, closed my eyes, and waited, and waited, and—

Bam.

Unbelievable. My brothers shook their heads, convinced I was adopted. Dad must have also considered the possibility. If Mom witnessed this magnetic display of ball-to-head, I'm sure she would have too.

Dad never took me seriously after that, yet I continued to play baseball every spring. He showed up every once in a while, always unannounced, always far from the other parents, and when I spotted him, I always screwed up by making an error or striking out.

At one of his surprise appearances, the umpire didn't show, so Dad volunteered. Since no one knew he was my father, no one objected—no one but me.

Mum's the word.

I had an uneventful game, but I had a chance to be the hero in the final inning. I stood at the plate with the go-ahead run at second. I worked the count to full: three balls, two strikes. A walk would extend the game, but a hit would win it. As I waited for the payoff pitch, my focus bounced back and forth between the pitcher forty-six feet in front of me and the home plate umpire crouched six feet behind. The pitcher wound up and delivered. I held up as the ball sailed high and outside. Clearly ball four.

Yet I heard, "Strike three, you're out."

I dropped my bat and hung my head. The opposing team rushed the mound and cheered, "Two, four, six, eight, who do we appreciate . . ." That game forever cemented my baseball relationship with my father. He never came to another game, and we never discussed it until years later when I included it in a gift of seventy-five memories for his seventy-fifth birthday. Most memories were happy, some were pithy, but I cherished them all. Dad said he remembered that game and admitted the ball was high and outside, definitely not a strike.

"But I taught you to never go down without swinging," he added. Then he stunned me when he said, "I've regretted that call for twenty-three years."

Twenty-three years. How we wasted all that time in between. Fuck mum's the word.

Mom saw a few of my good games, and though her attempts were futile, she always defended me to Dad. Despite my inauspicious beginnings, I became a good ballplayer. At fourteen, I led the league in home runs, made the All-Star team, and had a game of all games. I batted four for four with back-to-back-to-back home runs—two grand slams and a three-runner—and I drove in two more runs for good measure on my last trip to the plate. Thirteen runs in one game. *Thirteen*. Only major leaguer Wilbert Robinson came close when he drove in eleven for the Baltimore Orioles in 1892.

When I told my dad, he replied, "You're full of soup." He didn't believe me. Realizing I would never gain his respect through baseball, I gave it up.

Even though we never got it together on the field, ironically, baseball kept us close. When we didn't go to Yankee Stadium, we watched the Yankees play on TV or listened to their games on the radio. When he came to visit me during my college years at Ohio State, we went to the Clippers games, the Yankees' Triple-A farm team based in Columbus. On the day Mickey Mantle died, I felt the need to call my dad, and we shared stories.

During my father's last week on earth, we bet our usual one dollar on the World Series. His team won, but unfortunately, he never got the chance to collect his winnings.

The first time I saw *Field of Dreams*, I cried at the end when the main character asked his estranged father to play catch. The entire film had been building up to that "If you build it, he will come" moment when father and son finally came together. I took my father to see it long past its opening, hoping he, too, would be moved. We sat in the nearly empty Egyptian Theater in Hollywood. As that scene rolled, I saw through my teary eyes my dad wiping away tears of his own.

I hope one day we get a second chance to play catch. I can always dream.

CHAPTER 17

The Best Medicine

While sipping her early morning juice,
Mom turns to me with furrowed brow.

Mom: I call you all the time. Why don't you
call me?

Me: You call me. I come running. I call you.
What are you going to do?

Mom: (shrugging) I don't know.

In April, Deecy returned with her entire family and again pitched in taking care of Mom. After a few days, we needed a break. Michael suggested a hike in the mountains in upstate New York might be the ticket. We left Mom in the capable hands of yet another new hospice nurse and took off to commune with nature for a couple of hours.

When we returned, an overzealous Tweedle Dumb greeted us at the front door. "You're not going to believe this." She was way too happy for this to be bad news, but still her curious joy gave me pause.

We entered the kitchen and found Mom at the table, sitting in a wheelchair with the nurse by her side. At first, I was pissed that yet another one had ignored her supervisor's directive, "Keep her in bed."

And where did the wheelchair come from?

Sensing my anger, the nurse chimed in, "I took one look at your mother and said this lady is not ready to die. You are getting out of bed and into the kitchen to eat your lunch."

I watched in amazement as Mom fed herself for the first time since this whole thing began. She seemed content, even happy. Serious doubts about hospice crept in. They meant well, but their initial assessment was wrong. Her body wasn't shutting down. Food was necessary. And though Mom's performance in February might have been Oscar-worthy, she wasn't ready to die. This rebel nurse assessed her patient and prescribed the best medicine of all: common sense. From that day forward, I did too.

CHAPTER 18

Odd Jobs and Early Investments

One day, Mom and her red motorized reclining chair
were just about vertical.

Me: Where do you think you're going?

Mom: I've got to go to work.

Me: How are you going to get there?

Mom: I'll drive.

Me: Mom, you haven't worked in twenty years,
and you haven't driven in ten.

As far back as I can remember, the Porro kids worked. In the early days, the boys mowed lawns, raked leaves, shoveled snow, and delivered newspapers. With few options back then, the girls babysat or taught ballet in our basement. In addition to making my parents' bed for twenty-five cents, I went door to door selling old bleach bottles filled with sand from our crawl space as a get-your-stuck-car-out-of-the-snow miracle worker. I also hawked old newspapers—my own entrepreneurial idea—and, to my delight, actually made some sales, though I think more for my neighbor's amusement. The sand at least had a practical purpose. The old newspapers, not so much.

Our paper routes were extensive and had to be completed by the start of school. So, after returning home from working all night at *The Record*, Mom would wrestle each of us out of bed in shifts: first Michael, then David, and then me. She would then drive us on our designated routes until we delivered every last paper. Our mother endured this torture for years and without complaint.

Though we kept busy on our own, Mom kept us even busier. In the winter, we sold boxes of personalized Christmas cards, and wreaths in three sizes. In the summer, we delivered thick, heavy phone books, as well as samples of new products like Gain laundry detergent. Taking two of us at a time, we hopped on and off the open tailgate of our Dodge station wagon with the goods and back again as Mom drove at a snail's pace down each street. We worked nonstop until the car was empty.

But our smooth operation had a hiccup one day. After completing deliveries, Caryl and I collapsed in the back of the car, our weary legs dangling off the tailgate. As we headed home, Mom sped up just as I leaned forward to rub my sore feet, and I somersaulted out and onto the street. Luckily, no cars trailed close behind. That would have been messy.

Dazed, confused, and reeling in pain, I heard Caryl beckoning, "Come on, come on, come on." Her voice was a whisper, but her hands screamed, "Get back in this car before Mom finds out or we'll both be in trouble."

I struggled to my feet and staggered after the car. I caught up with it and dove in when Mom stopped at the next intersection. Caryl shielded my bruised, battered, and bloody body from Mom's rearview mirror check.

"Everything all right?"

We answered with an emphatic "yes." I winced while suppressing a painful giggle. After making sure my injuries weren't life threatening, Caryl giggled too. A close call, but we escaped, or thought we had. When Mom discovered my torn and bloody clothes buried under the laundry pile, we had to come clean, and our days of hanging off the tailgate ended.

The money earned from those odd jobs, along with our birthday checks, contributed to our first bank accounts at the Imperial Bank in Ridgewood. To get children excited about saving, they filled a sandbox with pennies, and we had one minute to stuff as many as we could into a plastic piggy bank emblazoned with their logo. I was hooked. We got our own bank books, but as kids we had little control over the funds. As our savings grew, Mom withdrew them and bought shares of Union Oil. When I first heard, I accused her of stealing my hard-earned cash.

How dare she buy stocks without discussing it with me, her ten-year-old son.

I got over it, but I didn't fully appreciate the value of investing until some thirty years later.

CHAPTER 19

A Whole New Ballgame

(Mom tenses up as soon as I enter.)

Me: Sorry, did I scare you?

Mom: Yes.

Me: I never want to scare you.

(She puckers up for a kiss.)

Me: Is that what this was all about?

(She shoots me a wicked smile.)

Life was never the same once Mom decided to wake up. There would be no more shoes, no more standing, no more walking, no more showers, no more going to the toilet on her own. The only daily activities she could manage without help were sitting, sleeping, and finding the Animal Planet channel with the TV remote. The rest was up to us, but mostly it was up to me. She had no qualms about having her every need met, and I do mean her every need. We all put up with it, some out of duty, but I found joy in it.

Deecy and I shared the tips and tricks we learned from hospice with Michael and Laurel. David and Caryl chose to be hands-off, but they contributed in other ways. To be honest, the fewer Porros the better when tackling any challenge. Whether or not intentional, our parents raised six strong-willed, stubborn, independent children.

After meeting us for the first time, Deecy's husband-to-be, a soft-spoken Michigan man we called Big Mike, remarked, "The Porros all have opinions, and they don't mind sharing them."

My response to him was: "We're from Jersey. Get over it."

Some say people from New Jersey are bold, some would even call us—dare I say it—brash, but Big Mike was right. Each of us had our own way of doing things. Each of us knew better. And if you put more than one of us in a room to complete a task, friction inevitably ensued.

Despite that, we trusted each other with Mom's care, though some handled the tender-loving part better than others.

My care routine went something like this:

Fill a bucket with warm, soapy water.

Wake Mom by ten if she's not already up.

Lower the bed rail and give her a kiss.

Wrestle the stuffed animals from her clutches with a combination of charm and muscle.

Deal with the likely separation anxiety.

Once calm has been restored, set her toys on the loveseat next to her bed where they would be in clear view.

Power the head of the bed down until flat.

Support her back while lifting under her knees, and rotate her so she's perpendicular to the bed.

Sit her up.

Loosen the diaper tabs.

Ask her to put her arms around my waist.

When she does, I place my hands under her armpits and start the countdown to make sure we're in sync: "One, two, three, up."

With her assisting as best she can, slowly stand her up.

Now, it would be a wonder if I got Mom from the bed to the commode—three feet away—without a stream of pee tracing every inch of our path. *Was that too much to ask?* Most mornings, yes.

So, keep her loosened diaper on for the three-foot journey.

Rotate her toward the commode.

Ask her to jiggle her hips so the diaper drops.

As usual, it lands with a soggy thud.

"One, two, three, and . . ."

Slowly lower her onto the commode.

Discard the wet diaper then don sterile gloves.

Mom removes her dentures and hands them to me to clean. She didn't like anyone seeing her without them, but when I told her she looked cute, she gave me a dirty look and pinched my nose. She's from Missour-uh all right.

Brush her teeth, then hand her a cup of mouthwash and a spit tray.

Have her rinse her mouth twice.

Mom resists the second swill. "For God's sake, it's not castor oil. It's pleasant-tasting Cool Mint Listerine."

She finally concedes after my pleading and cajoling.

After she finishes her business on the commode, often accompanied by color commentary—"I peed five big ones and two little drips!"—position the walker in front of her. "Mom, grab the handles."

I go behind to assist, once again, placing my hands under her armpits. "One, two, three, up."

Lift her to a standing position.

She steadies herself with the walker. Her arms and legs are remarkably stable for her age and lack of activity.

I quickly, yet meticulously, clean her butt with a warm, wet, soapy washcloth.

When done, help shuffle her to the bed. She sits on the edge with her feet flat on the floor.

I set my foot against hers so she doesn't slide off (not that this ever happened, *more than once.*)

Remove her nightgown and lay her down for a sponge bath.

Wash her front, gently roll her onto her right side and wash her back, then do the same on the left side.

Apply body lotion, deodorant, lip balm, then Balmex on her privates to help prevent diaper rash.

Sprinkle baby powder, roll her again, place a new adult diaper under her, add a feminine pad for extra absorption, then roll her back and secure the diaper.

Sit her up using the same method as before, and always with the countdown.

Let her choose her wardrobe, which includes a fresh day dress, clean socks, and depending on the weather, leggings, sweater, and gloves.

Brush her hair and secure it in a ponytail with a scrunchie.

Position the wheelchair next to the bed. The first time I turned away to get the wheelchair, she flopped back down because she didn't have any core strength. Fortunately, she didn't get hurt, but from then on, I placed the wheelchair close and locked the wheels before sitting her up. (Trust me, secure the wheels—not that it ever rolled away when she tried to sit down on it, *more than once*.)

"One, two, three, up." Lift, rotate, and slowly lower her into the wheelchair.

Place her feet on the footrests. If she's cold, place a blanket on her lap.

In the days that followed, we added personal touches that became favorites. We gave each other a morning hug, and when I pressed my forehead to hers, she let out a soft hum, and I answered with my own. We kept our foreheads together to see who could hum the longest. Sometimes I'd let her win, but not always. That girl could hum, though it shouldn't have been a surprise. She had lots of practice. During family dinners, she often ended her sentences with a hum.

"Please pass the salad, hmm."

"Ridgewood sidewalk sales start tomorrow, hmm."

When I called her out, she, of course, denied it. And because she just couldn't control herself, she punctuated her denial with a hum that sent us all into hysterics, including the hum-meister herself.

Back to the routine.

Once mobile, wheel her into the vestibule so she can check on the weather and any neighborhood activities before heading to the kitchen for breakfast.

"Hands up," I say.

She raises them to avoid getting pinched by the table as we roll around it (not that this ever happened either, *more than once*. It's a learning process. I'm a first-time parent. Give me a break.)

Place a bib on her and allow her time to greet each of her porcelain figurines: Zuri, the praying angel, and Santa. Yes, Santa, year-round.

Before breakfast, serve Mom daily doses of Ensure and Pro-Stat protein drinks to keep up her strength.

After a lovely meal, roll her into the living room and lock the wheels.

"One, two, three, up." Lift, rotate, and slowly lower her onto the red reclining chair so she can watch television and take her inevitable nap before dinner.

If she's cold, cover her with Caryl's hand-made reversible blanket with built-in pockets —St. Patrick's Day on one side, St. Valentine's Day on the other.

While she sleeps, I clean commode, change bedding, dispose of the trash.

At six o'clock, I wheel her into the kitchen for dinner. Afterward, it's back to the living room for *Wheel of Fortune* and *Jeopardy* or to bed. Her choice.

Reverse the routine at night. However, this presented a different challenge: making sure she finished her business on the commode before I washed and readied her for bed. Mom had little control over what, where, or when things decided to leave her body . . . or on whom. My baptism happened one night just as I was about to secure a fresh diaper.

"Oh no, why now?"

Mom smiled. "It's natural."

It was bound to happen sooner or later. Images of a young mother getting peed on while changing her baby's diaper are adorable. But not if it's your mom. I wanted to cry but instead I laughed. She seemed to be fine with it, so I had to be as well.

Once comfortable in bed, place a pillow under her legs to elevate her feet. This prevents sores on her heels.

Return her stuffed animals one by one. She'll arrange them to her liking.

Finish with a goodnight kiss and a "Sweet dreams."

Lights off.

It's imperative to be encouraging, gentle, and to explain each step beforehand. No surprises. Though she sometimes had one for me, like tooting while I was cleaning her no-fly zone.

"Not nice, Mom."

But she apologized. One day, I accidentally paid her back. While making the bed with her in it—at times necessary—I covered her head with the top sheet. After pulling it down, I said, "Sorry, too soon?"

Need I remind you that a sense of humor is necessary, no matter how dark?

After seeing Mom's steady progress and knowing hospice was on board for a few more weeks, I felt comfortable enough to return to my snack-food business in Los Angeles. But knowing Tammy and the Tweedles would soon be back in charge caused me great concern. I believed they were partly responsible for Mom's death wish in February. And now she was even more dependent on them.

Mom and I kept in touch by phone until Michael introduced her and himself to the twenty-first century with iPads. FaceTime became our preferred form of communication. And despite the presence of Tammy and the Tweedles, Mom continued to do well. She looked good, her spirits remained high, and my concern eased . . . somewhat.

CHAPTER 20

Full Circle

Me: Good morning. How are you doing?
Mom: Happy couple.
Me: Happy couple? Who's your partner?
Mom: He scattered. Not so happy, after all.

It was October 1997. My visit was supposed to be a surprise but when I arrived, my father had one for me. The last time I saw him was at our summer family reunion. When we hugged goodbye, he—in the final throes of a seven-year battle with heart disease—whispered, "I don't think I'm long for this world."

I squeezed him tight and burst into tears. This time I wasn't alone. Seeing Dad cry was a rare event, but less so those days.

He wiped his eyes. "You know, we've got about an hour and a half of material here, but you already used it up in your screenplay."

Earlier in the week, I read aloud *Ritornare*, a tale inspired by our trip to Celle San Vito, Italy two years ago. Dad always sought the humor in things and often struck a bullseye. And even through all the waterworks, he did it again.

I returned to Los Angeles. Two months later, Michael called. "The doctor says he's got thirty days."

Reality struck. My mind froze. My stomach churned.

"Mark, are you there?"

"Yeah, yeah, got it. I'm coming home." I packed my navy-blue suit. Didn't want to bring black. Didn't want to wave the white flag at the inevitable. I wasn't ready for that. None of us were. I took the red-eye and landed in New Jersey at dawn.

As I walked up my parents' driveway, I noticed the side door was ajar, which was strange this time of year. My father made sure to never waste utilities. We kids often heard comments like, "Are we heating the entire neighborhood too?" He'd even turn off the lights before I reached the top of the steps.

I pushed the door open and peeked inside. There was a red trail from the stove to my father's bloody foot on the black-and-white tiles. I crept in, not wanting to disturb the scene. Perhaps I played too many detective roles. He was lying face up, his eyes closed, his body still. *Jesus Christ*. Moments ago, I'd debated whether to have breakfast before heading over. Now I found my father dead on the kitchen floor.

"Dad?" I whispered.

No response.

This time louder, "Dad."

His eyes snapped open. I jumped. "Marky Brother, what the heck are you doing here?"

Relieved, I said, "Oh, I just happened to be in the neighborhood. What are you doing down there?"

He shrugged. "I fell off that darn thing and can't get up." A poor excuse for a rolling chair sat next to him. Outmatched at his normal one hundred and sixty-five pounds. The extra forty of water weight from congestive heart failure made this mobility choice dangerous. But as stubborn as all get-out, and not at all content when confined in bed, he took a chance.

"You cut your foot."

"Yeah? Don't feel a thing."

I sat him up. After he caught a few quick breaths—deep ones were no longer possible—we plodded back to his room and back to the safety of his hospital bed. "Where's Mom?"

He chuckled. "Out shopping. No telling how long she'll be."

In 1975, during my freshman year at college, Mom's shopping addiction and weight gain hit a critical stage. On Christmas break, I tried to find out why. When my naturally chatty mother refused to talk, I resorted to extreme measures. Under false pretenses—and in the eyes of the law could only be considered kidnapping—I drove her to the Duck Pond in the dead of winter and promised, "Neither of us is getting back in the car until you tell me what's going on."

But be careful what you wish for. After an hour in the bitter cold, her impenetrable emotional armor melted.

"This is not how a husband should treat his wife!" she cried out.

Her admission stunned me. What followed broke my heart. She shared for the first time some of the cruel things my father had called her, and her overall disappointment in their marriage.

I grew up with the friction. When you put two flinty personalities together, you're bound to spark some. At times, Dad's sharp tongue shook the house, and Mom's defiance brought out the worst in him. Tensions escalated when she ignored his objections and bought my brother David a puppy. We had lots of cats and other furry creatures over the years, but no dog until Shadow entered the picture. He was known as "The Casanova of Emmett Place" until his overactive libido burned out sixteen years later. My parents' marriage hit the tipping point when she defied him yet again by keeping a puppy my sister Caryl rescued from certain death at the hands of drunk teenagers. And though Dad often threatened divorce, he admitted they couldn't afford it.

But in the heat of all their arguments, the only insult I heard Dad hurl at Mom was "gold digger," which I found amusing. She was not only emotionally independent but financially as well. She had a good-paying job, bought her own clothes, her own car, and much of the food.

In fact, Mom provided the down payment on our home.

In 1970, after Caryl's tearful plea to go to marriage counseling, they did. I saw little change in my mother. My father, no pushover himself, at least tried to apply what he'd learned. For Mother's Day, he bought Mom a basket full of beauty products. I remember thinking, *What are you trying to tell her?*

But Dad went shopping for Mom. That alone was amazing. Usually, he would just hand her a check. However, on their first post-counseling trip, when Mom dashed all hope of rekindling any romance by refusing to remove her girdle, Dad gave up. When he shared this with me during his coast-to-coast retirement trip in 1985, we had the sex talk—with *me* coaching *him*.

The only sex advice he ever gave me was well into my twenties after I introduced him to my first serious girlfriend.

"Let the girl set the pace," he said.

Mom's only advice? "No sex before marriage. No if, ands, or buts." And she never wavered.

When coaching my dad, I asked, "Were you a caring and generous lover?"

He felt he was.

That broke the ice. We discussed everything: their first date, their marriage, their money issues. When Mom spent much of the honeymoon shopping, he felt the marriage was a mistake. Three decades and six kids later, what do you say to that? But his honesty and vulnerability blew me away. I no longer saw my father as the "bad guy." My mother shared equal blame in that drama.

To sustain the marriage, they lived on separate floors and often took separate vacations for years. And they, as good Catholics do, stuck it out. Only till death did they part.

When Mom retired, Caryl—hoping to bring some joy to the home—took a chance and gifted her a Bichon Frisé puppy. Zuri became Mom's seventh and, one could argue, favorite child.

Dad surprised us all by welcoming the newest member of the family. I once caught him petting the pup under the table and whispering, "Good doggy, good doggy."

But Zuri's healing powers only went so far. Mom and Dad continued to sleep on separate floors.

We witnessed a reconciliation of sorts during Dad's final years. Mom stuck by his side. They worked as a team to battle his heart disease and became nearly inseparable. Dad confirmed this by signing his typewritten updates with a combination of their names, *Genoel*.

Mom was the main reason he stayed at home instead of in the hospital, as per his wish. But that decision required an extraordinary effort on her part. No spring chicken herself, she struggled to get him in and out of the house, and to and from the outpatient heart clinic several times a week. When Caryl witnessed our seventy-six-year-old mother crouch behind our eighty-two-year-old father and push his butt up the four steps to the house, she begged them to move to the Jersey Shore so she could take care of them.

Mom had smiled at Dad. "We're doing all right, aren't we?"

He nodded yes, and our iron-willed parents stayed put.

I witnessed this tandem perform their stair-climbing technique just once. Even though it was painful to watch, it was a beautiful sight to see.

Mom's sacrifice and commitment, heroic by any measure, was appreciated by us all, but none more than Dad. His eyes lit up whenever she entered the room, and his hand always reached out to meet hers. Kisses between the two had become the new norm.

Three days before he left this world, Mom floated into the kitchen after spending a few minutes alone with Dad, her face all aglow.

"What happened?" I asked.

She grinned. "He said I have a good heart." And just like that, any lingering bitterness from their forty-nine-year marriage simply vanished. "He doesn't want to be buried alone, so I said, 'Okay, I'll join ya.'"

They had broken their long-standing vow to spend their eternal lives in separate graves. From that moment on, I don't believe my mother uttered a negative word about my father or their marriage. In a sense, they came full circle.

CHAPTER 21

Better Than Food

(Mom wakes up all peppy. She waves
her finger at me.)

Mom: I have not had one glass of water
since I've been here.

(I return with a glass. She guzzles it.)

Mom: You're supposed to drink eight glasses a day.

Me: Well, you've got seven more to go.

Mom: (dismissing me with a wave) No thanks.

Aside from my father's corny jokes and avoiding Mom's shopping marathons, most of our family traditions revolved around food. Dad was clever. He hid his lack of culinary skills by entertaining the troops. His show magically made everything he cooked up taste better. When serving his creations, he often proclaimed them "better than food." And who were we to disagree?

His crazy-shaped pancakes always delighted, as did his orange, olive, and maraschino cherry salad—even with those salty anchovies mixed in. Dad roasted chestnuts all year long, and could satisfy the six of us with a single pomegranate. His made-from-leftovers spaghetti sauces and soups—which he called "Baseball Zoup" during baseball season—were weekly staples. He introduced us to lentils, but also liver and onions (yuck). He made an art out of taking day-old corn on the cob, peeling off one row at a time, distributing whole kernels into our eager hands. All that was left was a perfectly clean cob, which, of course, went right into the compost heap. He stuffed ice cream cones with cold mashed potatoes that never melted on a sweltering summer day. We all joined in on the Coconut Toss, where we threw one, drained of its juices, down the basement steps until we heard that magical sound—*crack!* It didn't take long after for us to stuff ourselves silly with every morsel of white meat.

Mom didn't need a show. While she was no Julia Child in the kitchen, she did excel at baking.

One of my favorites was her "still-the-best-lasagna-ever." Her cherry, apple, and pumpkin pies always melted in your mouth, warmed your stomach, and made every holiday much better. Her vast array of Christmas cookies could put any Michelin-starred pastry chef to shame. They were all so good that even when I held my hand high above my head and declared, "I'm filled up to here," I always managed to stuff in another one, or two, or three. I still have fond yet foggy memories of getting tipsy testing her terrible-tasting Whiskey Balls (say that three times fast, and then try it after a few Whiskey Balls).

In 1963, Dad introduced us to something unique and truly special, his half-popped popcorn snack he called "Nutra Nuts." And a new family tradition was born. His motivation, in part, was his fear of impending dental bills since all his children inherited in various degrees his sweet tooth. Hoping to protect his wallet and our teeth, he set out to invent a snack, healthier and yet as addicting as that darn candy.

How he came up with the idea remains a mystery—not a *mum's the word* mystery, but a genuine mystery. How he achieved success was not. He spent hours experimenting in his lab, Mom's kitchen. He customized her pots. He splattered hot oil all over and filled the house with fumes night after night until he came up with these crunchy golden nuggets packed with corn flavor. But Dad wasn't done yet. For extra protein, he mixed in roasted soy nuts decades before they became popular in the US. He added a pinch of salt, and voilà: Nutra Nuts.

Friends and family couldn't get enough of them. But after years of attempts to acquire a patent or to sell the secret process failed, Dad grew disenchanted with the whole idea. By the early eighties, he gave up on his dream entirely. Only Mom's kitchen was happy about it.

In 1992, during our third family reunion, the story of Nutra Nuts came up. I thought how sad it was that my nieces and nephews never got a chance to taste their Grandpa Po's snack. I always had a passion for Nutra Nuts. I assisted Dad many times in the kitchen and often spent my days at Our Lady of Mount Carmel, drawing plans for the future Nutra Nuts factory.

When I returned to Los Angeles, I called Dad and told him, "I'm reviving Nutra Nuts. Please give me the secret formula."

He did, and though I cannot share the "how," I can tell you that it is a messy, and at times dangerous, process. You must protect yourself with goggles, a hat, an oil-resistant apron, and oven mitts. Still, I nearly burned down my studio apartment and died by asphyxiation.

But Nutra Nuts were reborn and quickly devoured. I risked another fire, made more, and brought a batch with me to the next family reunion. My dad's smile made my near-death experience worth it. The family gobbled them up in no time, just like we did so many years ago.

My family's response, along with my friends and contacts in Hollywood, convinced me it was time to share Nutra Nuts with the world. With Dad's approval, I began researching the industry, attending trade shows, and visiting stores. There was still nothing like it out there on the market. The timing in the midnineties was perfect. The soy craze was just beginning, and since organic snacks were becoming popular, I went organic with Nutra Nuts. I shared logo and packaging designs with my dad for his input. He only asked that his image not be used.

But before Nutra Nuts became a reality, my father died. One year later, in 1998, Michael and I founded the Better Than Food company to honor him. Dad didn't want his image used, but I wanted his name on every bag, so Grandpa Po's Originals replaced Nutra Nuts. This also eliminated confusion in the marketplace since there were no actual nuts in it. We first introduced Dad's original flavor, Slightly Unsalted—his play on words—and we added Slightly Spicy and Slightly Sweet soon after. Within a few years, we grew his snack into a national brand.

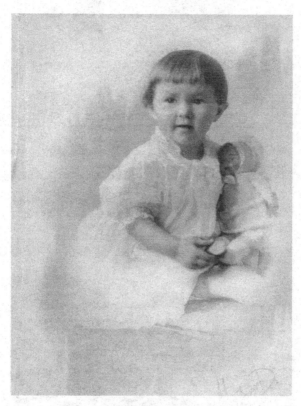

Genevieve Mary Brennan at
eighteen months old

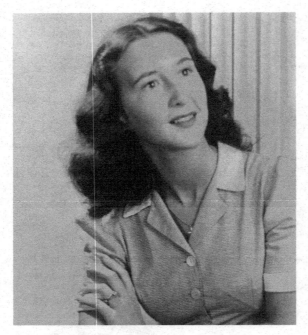

Genevieve the hand model

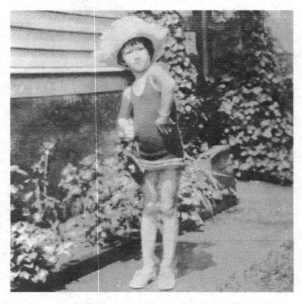

Spunky Genevieve

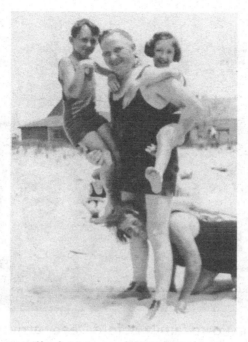

John, Wilhelmina and Genevieve Brennan
at the beach with a cousin

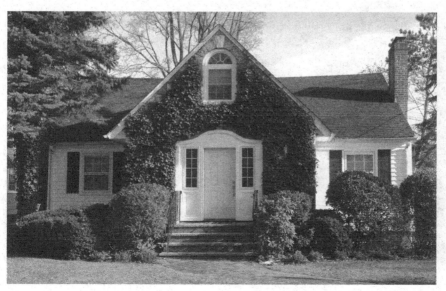

247 Emmett Place (2014)

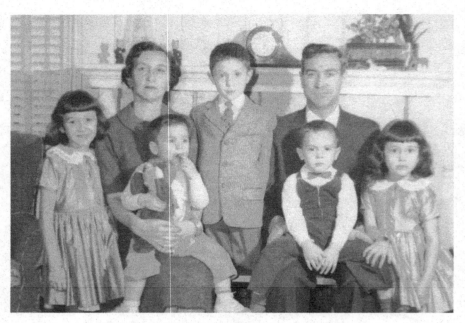

The Porro family before Deecy arrived

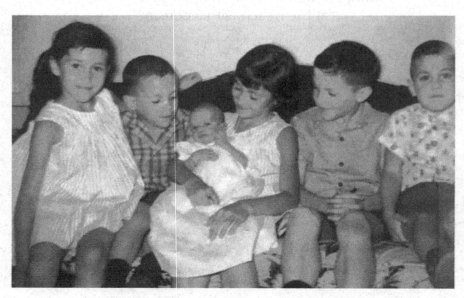

The five Porro kids welcome Deecy

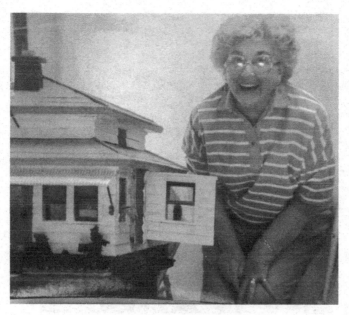

Uncle William's refurbished dollhouse
pleases Mom to no end

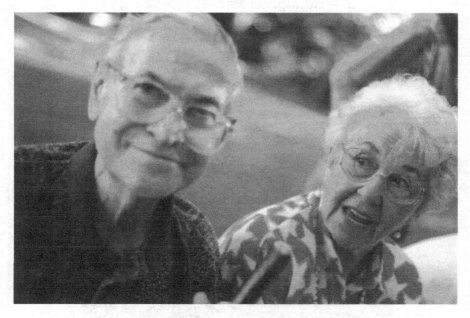

Dad's last family reunion (August 1997)

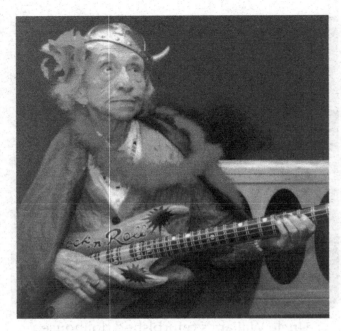

Mom's shows off her goofy side at granddaughter Rachel's wedding

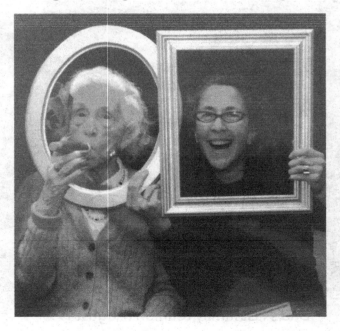

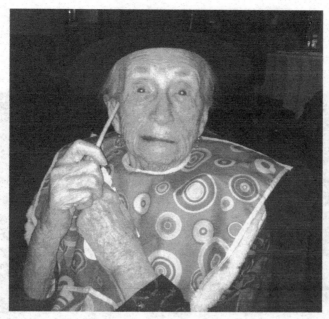

A breadstick Genevieve couldn't refuse

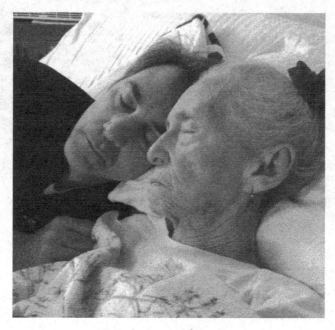

Our journey begins

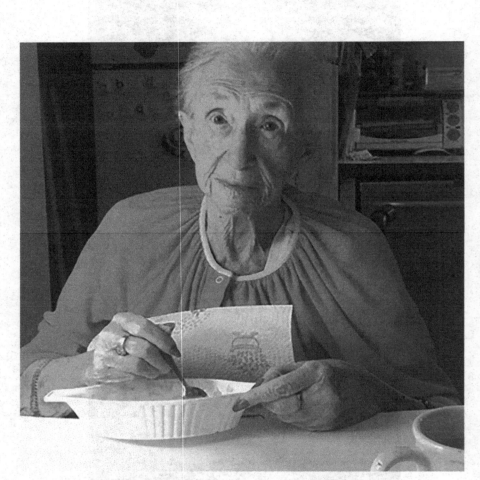

No medicines, no problem, I've got sherbet.
Bowls and bowls of sherbet.

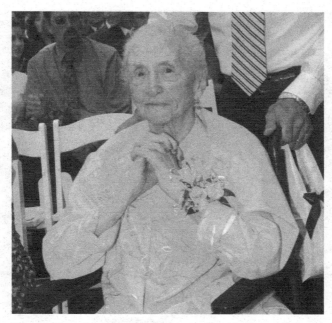

Mom almost stole the show at Josh and Maggie's wedding

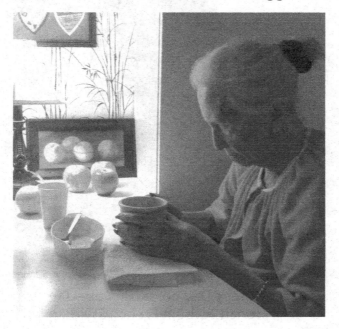

Quiet time to sit, reflect, and enjoy a cup of tea

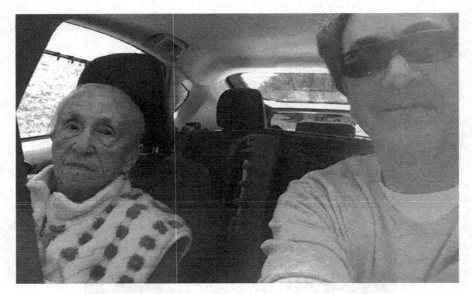

Gallivanting

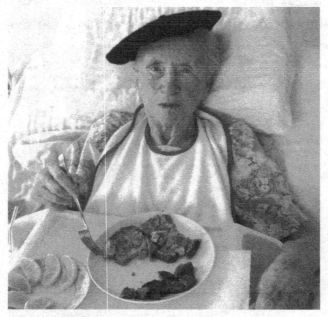

Mother's Day breakfast in bed.
French Toast in French Style

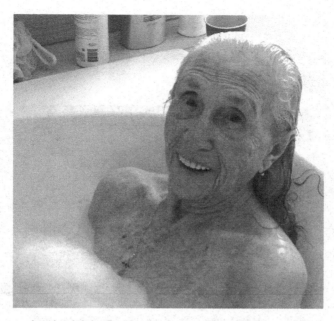

The bubble bath that was almost her last.
At least she smelled good

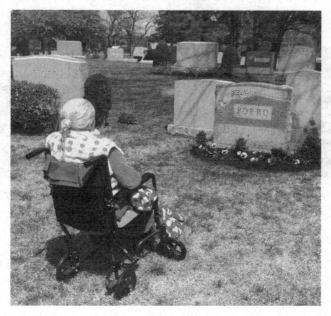

Visiting Dad when she whispered 'I miss ya'

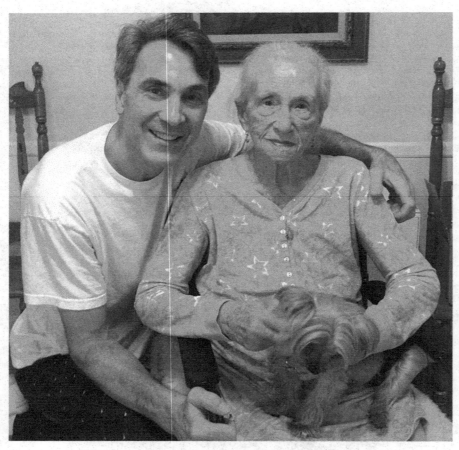

Just out of the hospital. Twenty pounds lighter
but ready to get back to work

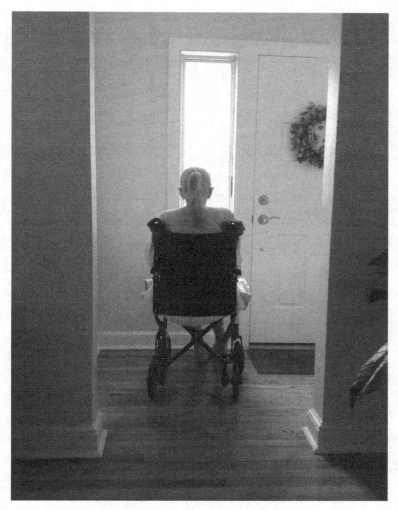

Before breakfast, Mom checks on
what's going on outside.

CHAPTER 22

It Might Be Time to Get Mom Some Help

Why not? It's convenient. —Mom

In 2006, when Mom turned eighty-four, she began falling, *a lot*. She hadn't broken a hip yet, but it was only a matter of time. She wanted to stay home with Zuri, and since Mom and her walker had not yet bonded, we needed to hire live-in help. Having someone keeping an eye on her gave us all peace of mind. In addition to helping Mom stay on her feet and off the floor, she needed help cooking meals, cleaning house, and doing laundry.

To prepare the house for our new guests, I flew in from the "Left Coast," as Dad called it, to do the much-needed repairs. Mom's perpetually peeing pooch rendered every inch of the wall-to-wall carpeting a health hazard, making its removal a priority. Hidden under years of plush cream, textured gold, and green shag, I found a delightful surprise: a beautiful hardwood floor begging to be born again. After heavy sanding and a light coat of shellac, its new pee-proof life began. I installed a working shower in the upstairs bathroom. The previous one was nothing more than a closet for Mom's bargains. After a few final touches and a fresh coat of paint, the house was ready.

Michael placed an ad in the local papers: "Seeking an individual or a family to provide meals, laundry, cleaning, and companionship for our mother in exchange for rent and utilities in a pleasant house on a quiet cul-de-sac in a lovely village with an excellent education system." Who could resist?

Before help arrived, I asked my mother about the many patches of dead grass peppering the backyard. She gleefully admitted that she and Zuri pee together. "Why not? It's convenient."

Believing we hit a new low in human-dog "togetherness," I asked, "What about the neighbors?"

She shrugged. "They can't see anything. I'm in my night-dress."

"Without your panties, I hope."

"Of course. I just spread my legs a little and let it go."

First, too much information, and second, this didn't help matters. I considered adding lawncare to the list of duties while we still had one.

Mona, a nurse's aide at the Valley Hospital just four blocks away, was the first to try her hand. This seemed like a good fit until she realized the job involved real work. Mom could be difficult, especially if her "I'm-from-Missour-uh" bullshit detector went off. With Mona it redlined, making Mom nearly impossible to please. Mona had issues, and they only added to her difficulties at 247. She refused to marry the immigrant father of her three-year-old daughter, believing he only wanted to get married to gain his citizenship. She, in turn, aimed her bitterness at the little girl and at Mom. Mona's love of Clorox smacked of work—a habit she no doubt picked up from the hospital—but when the nose-hair-curling fog lifted, there was little evidence of any actual cleaning.

After observing Mona's neglect during one of my visits, I politely asked, "Can you please tell me what you do here?"

"I don't have time for this," she snapped. "I got to take care of my kid." She then slammed a McDonald's cheeseburger down on the kitchen table and stormed out, leaving her daughter alone with me. Her definition of "taking care of her kid" was my next question, but I didn't get the chance to ask it.

The last straw came when Mona accused Mom of trying to strangle her. Michael asked, "What could you have possibly done to so anger an eighty-four-year-old lady?"

Mona was outraged. "I knew you'd take her side," she fired back.

Of course he did. This was not a *Sophie's Choice*, even for my Brother Teresa, who more often than not gave the guilty the benefit of the doubt.

Gone but not forgotten, Mona left the entire contents of her deceased father's house in our basement, where it stayed for many years. Her loss was the Salvation Army's gain. Our experience with Mona prompted an additional question for the next candidate: "Are you, or does anyone else think you are batshit crazy?"

Our second team, Sally and Mariano, were anything but. This delightful couple genuinely loved life, their job, and our mother. Sally was a nurse. Mariano was a personal aide and handyman. There couldn't have been a better combination for Mom. They kept her and the house in tip-top shape. Unfortunately, after a year, they saved up enough money to buy their own home and off they went.

Sally and Mariano's departure opened the door for the Tweedles, who arrived in 2008.

CHAPTER 23

It's Like Déjà Vu All over Again

*Tweedle Dumb: Why don't you go back
to California?
We were all fine before you came.
Me: Of course you were. Until you got caught.*

Several weeks after returning to Los Angeles, someone, I don't remember who, emailed me a photo more disturbing than Aunt Claire's postmortem prints. Mom sat alone in the living room, slumped in her wheelchair with a travel pillow jammed under her chin. I wasn't sure if she was dead or alive. Who would think *that* image would bring me comfort? Or was *that* the idea? So, when I returned in September for a family wedding, I was not surprised to find little had changed at 247 Emmett Place.

Dust once again covered every surface and cobwebs clung to every corner. Grain moths, now in even greater numbers, flew in battle formation, spying the lone obstacle between them and the bounty of open food on the counters: an army of ants. Deecy and I had tackled the insect problem in February. We sealed all of the Tweedles' packages, and deep cleaned and disinfected all of the kitchen cabinets. We hoped to inspire them to do the same, but all we did was inspire them to watch.

The bedroom reeked of urine again. Sanitary gloves were nowhere to be found. Tammy ignored the hospice training and instead favored her own method of hoisting my mother in and out of bed. Mom grimaced while she held on for dear life as Tammy performed her Hulk Hogan-type move. It was painful to watch, and a miracle Mom escaped injury, but she was a good sport and never complained. Or was she afraid to?

At mealtime, the Tweedles continued to park Mom in the kitchen facing the wall while they scurried about, whispering behind her back, and paying no attention to the fact she heard most, if not all, of what they said.

The only welcome change was a hospital bed with an alternating pressure mattress. This enhanced Mom's circulation and helped prevent future bedsores. Other than that, like Yogi Berra said, "It was like déjà vu all over again." We were right back to where we started.

To keep my sanity, I took over all of Tammy's caregiving duties, and many of the Tweedles' chores too. But I also had to prepare for Mom's trip to her grandson Josh's wedding at the Jersey Shore. This would mark her first outing since her near-death experience back in February.

Getting her out of the house provided her a healthy break. The trip, however, presented its fair share of challenges. How would she handle the two-hour car ride, sleeping in a hotel bed, and sitting on a standard toilet? We would soon find out. I made a list and packed everything we needed for the weekend's events: clothes, medicine, makeup, lotions, bed pads, diapers, sanitary gloves, walker, wheelchair, tea, oatmeal, and her stuffed animals for bedtime. Check, check, and check. We zipped down the

Garden State Parkway and arrived with time to spare.

Drawing on my experience growing up with three sisters—I learned a lot more than how to put the toilet seat down—I took special care dolling Mom up on the day of the wedding. It was incredible to see what her favorite pink pantsuit, braided hair, bright-red lipstick, and nail polish could do for a lady, and to those around her. It brought back fond memories of her weekly pampering sessions at the beauty parlor.

Mom beamed as Abe, brother of the groom, rolled her down the garden aisle. She partook in all activities with gusto: gorging on the incredible variety of food, mugging for the camera in the photo booth, and swaying to the live music. At one point, forgetting she hadn't walked in eight months, Mom practically sprung from her wheelchair to join the others on the dance floor. Since tying her down wasn't a good look, we kept her seated and took turns partnering. Other than the bride and groom, Mom was the belle of the ball.

She looked so happy. I hadn't seen her smile like that in years. To keep her smiling, I realized

I had to play a bigger role in her care. When we returned home, I asked her if she wanted me to come back to make sure this level of care continued. She nodded yes.

But I wasn't sure how I was going to make that happen. I still had my snack business to run. I still had the occasional acting audition. I still had to support myself. Michael offered to hire me to redesign his offices. That solved one problem. The possibility of flying back and forth between coasts to keep my business alive solved another, but my acting career had to go.

So, goodbye Hollywood. Hello, New Jersey.

CHAPTER 24

Natale the Mayor

"Natale Porro, America 1891."
—Vito Cupola, Celle historian

T he story of my great-grandfather, Natale, and why he left Celle San Vito, Italy, in the 1890s, hung around our family's neck like an albatross. This wasn't the typical inspirational tale of a poor immigrant who came to America to seek a better life for his family. Far from it. Rumor had it that Natale, the mayor of Celle—a cool bit of history—was run out of town for committing adultery with his also-married secretary—not such a cool bit of history. I know what you're thinking. Italy of all places had an issue with infidelity? Apparently, yes. At least the villagers of Celle did. So, Natale fled to America.

The person who brought this tale across the Atlantic remains a mystery. What happened to mum's the word? At least Natale kept silent and did his best to outlive it. He died in 1951 at the age of ninety-six. But this dark chapter remained part of family lore until 1995.

That year, while working on a stage adaptation of Federico Fellini's 1963 classic film, *8½*, I got in touch with my inner Italian, which reignited my curiosity about my family history. I had a friend who boasted of his hero's welcome when he visited his grandfather's village in Italy. I wanted to experience that too. And despite my great-grandfather's peccadilloes, I took a chance on my own hero's welcome and planned a trip. It had been over a hundred years since Natale had been run out of town. What was the worst that could happen? I packed my running shoes just in case.

As a gift for his eightieth birthday, I invited Dad to join me, and after much prodding, he accepted. He was not a keen traveler. This would mark his first trip overseas. In World War II, he couldn't fly because of a chronic eardrum issue, which had also threatened his eligibility. Even after two rejections, he was determined to join the war effort. His third attempt was the charm. He enlisted as an army chemist but remained stateside in Utah, where he worked on things he didn't like talking about.

In 1995, flying was still a big deal for Dad, especially a long flight over the Atlantic. Another concern was his battle with congestive heart disease. Though it was gaining ground, he appeared to have it under control. It wasn't until I saw him stop at a curb in Rome and study its height, take a deep breath, then attempt to scale it did the severity of the disease he'd so bravely tried to hide become clear to me. I realized this trip would not be all fun and games. His life was literally in my hands. Whenever I offered to help, he snapped, "I'm not an invalid!" This became our routine, as did missing several buses, taxis, and trains.

Frustration was inevitable, and after yet another bus left us in the ancient Italian dust, he gasped, "Sorry for slowing us down."

"There's no need to apologize," I said after taking a deep breath of my own. "This is *your* trip. We'll go at *your* pace, and by doing so, we'll see *more* things." My reasoning seemed to ease his guilt, if only for the moment.

So, we slowed down, and we saw more things. Things that we might have otherwise missed. Unfortunately, that included ten extra hours of seeing more things. Our scheduled four-hour train ride turned into a fourteen-hour odyssey due to a combination of timesaving advice from well-meaning but uninformed passengers, my limited knowledge of the language, and our mobility issues. Desperate to end it, we agreed to get off at the next station, which left us in the middle of nowhere. The kind station manager took pity on us when he discovered we had no family, no friends, nor had any contact with anyone in Celle in over one hundred years. He drove us to a hotel in a nearby village to spend the night.

The next morning, we rented a car for the final leg and finally arrived in the quaint village of Celle San Vito, population two hundred. Three jovial ladies greeted us at the village gate. They spoke no English but tracked down Paolo who did . . . *somewhat*. With his bit of English and my bit of Italian, we understood each other enough to get by. I must admit, my spirited hands dominated every conversation and were much more successful than my words.

After explaining why we came, Paolo escorted us to the police station. Not a good sign. There he introduced us to Vito Cupola, the five-foot-three police chief, who was the entire police department and, by luck, Celle's village historian. Upon hearing that we were Americans, Vito launched into a soliloquy he enjoyed a *piccolo* too much. With his thick accent, I couldn't tell what it was about.

But to be safe, I turned to Dad and whispered, "Get ready to run."

He chuckled. "Easy for you to say."

We both knew running, or even walking at this point, was not an option. I steeled myself and offered up our family name.

Vito pounced. "Natale Porro, America, 1891."

Uh-oh, right on the tip of his tongue.

Paolo smiled. "He loves the tale of Natale the Mayor," he confessed. "He told it to me again just this morning."

Dad forced a polite smile.

I bristled. "Jesus, did nothing exciting happen in Celle since 1891?"

Celleans have been telling this story for over a century. But who told it to Vito? And who told the person who told Vito? And why? Comforted by the fact that we hadn't been run off yet, I asked Vito if I could film an encore performance of "The Tale of Natale the Mayor" while Paolo translated. Welcoming the opportunity, this one on camera, Vito took center stage.

"The mayor and his secretary were dallying. All the villagers knew but kept silent because they feared the powerful mayor."

Unfortunately, this confirmed the story we believed to be true.

Vito continued with soaring dramatic flair. "As word spread throughout the region, shame rained down on Celle, but still no one spoke up. Until one day, a courageous young man stormed into the mayor's office and demanded, 'You must stop this affair, or you must leave our village.' The mayor dismissed him with a laugh. But this young man's bravery galvanized the villagers into action. They rose up and ran both adulterers out of town. That brave young man was Natale."

I stared in disbelief. "Wait. What? Natale was the hero?"

Paolo and Vito nodded.

"But we heard Natale was the bad mayor."

"No, he *did this* to the bad mayor," Paolo reassured.

"Then why do you call him 'Natale the Mayor'?"

Paolo checked with Vito and then said, "He became the mayor after."

Finally, the real story. We cleared our family name, at least for those back in the States. Natale was as good as gold here. He didn't flee Celle San Vito in shame. He left to seek a better life for his family. His tale was indeed inspirational.

Vito then took us to Natale's house. It was unoccupied and closed up, but in the backyard, where no Porro had been in over a century, we found a pile of junk. Dad picked up a piece and said, "This must be why we don't throw out anything at home." Recycling is in our genes, passed down for generations. And though my sisters and I have done well in controlling those hereditary tendencies, my brothers have not been so lucky.

Though fruitful, our adventure was both physically and emotionally exhausting, especially for my father. But neither of us had any regrets. In fact, Dad admitted it was one of the highlights of his life. Mine too. We grew much closer during our sixteen days together, and I embraced my role as guardian. That experience would pay big dividends in the years to come.

CHAPTER 25

You Can Take the Kid Out of Jersey, But...

I'm the bully? I'm a kid. —Me

I don't know where I got my boldness. Certainly not from my dad. He avoided making waves or even ripples at all costs. Mom was a bit of a rebel. She insisted on walking my little sister down the aisle along with my father—a first, at least in our family. Maybe I got it from my great-grandfather, Natale, or from my two torture-loving brothers. Or perhaps I got it from where I grew up. In any case, if you mess with me, my family, my friends, or even a stranger, my "Jersey" comes out.

I had a theory about Hollywood. There was an exclusive club where the heavy hitters rubbed elbows and all big-time decisions were made.

To have any chance in this business, you had to get past the velvet rope and into that room. If you did, and if you had some talent, worked hard, and didn't screw up, things could go very well for you.

In the early nineties, I shared my theory with a "big-time" manager and closed with, "I believe you're the guy who can get me in. I'll take care of the rest."

He smiled and signed me on the spot. That weekend he invited me to a party at his house—impressive even by Hollywood standards. And to put a little cash in my pocket, he hired me to design and print new stationery, envelopes, and business cards for the office. I was on my way.

Two weeks later, I got a disturbing call from Mr. Big-Time's office.

"Come get your headshots and tapes."

"Why?" I asked as my stomach churned.

"They evicted him, repossessed his car, and cut off his phone."

Turned out Mr. Big-Time was a big-time conman. What made it worse was that he owed me for a $1,200 printing bill. He may have no longer needed the stationery, envelopes, and business cards, but I needed that money. Much to his surprise, I tracked him down. Charming as ever, he denied nothing, and even seemed amused by it all. Then he invited me to sue him in small claims court.

"But the line of creditors is long," he warned.

I sued and won, but nothing happened. A subsequent writ of execution to garnish his wages did no good because he had no wages to garnish. So I waited. He soon resurfaced at a mid-level talent agency. I called to congratulate him.

"Come in, I'll cut you a check," he said happily.

My mother was visiting from New Jersey, so I took her along. Mr. Big-Time wouldn't dare write a bad check in her presence. As soon as Mom laid eyes on him, she shot me her "I'm-from-Missour-uh" look. Taking no chances, I raced to his bank, check in hand. The account had been closed weeks ago. He *dared*.

They say the easiest person to con is a conman. I decided to test this theory.

Putting my theatrical skills to good use, I called his agency posing as the Beverly Hills Sheriff. Mr. Big-Time intercepted the call. He, having no idea I was on the other end, flat out lied. I played along, maintaining my cool as best I could until I hung up.

After a fair amount of venting, I called the owner of the agency, again introduced myself as the sheriff, and demanded, "Do not let him [Mr. Big-Time] on this call. He just lied to an officer of the law. I need your word he'll make good on what's owed to the plaintiff [me]."

He promised. And over the next few weeks, I recovered the full amount. I conned a conman and perhaps committed a felony of my own. I hope the statute of limitations applies here.

In the sixth grade, after an unsuccessful day of fishing at Collisie's Pond, my friend and I headed home. As we climbed up the wooded hill, boulders large enough to do serious damage suddenly rained down on us. We ducked behind trees to avoid injury. When the coast cleared, I snuck a peek and caught sight of two high schoolers laughing at the top of the hill, one I recognized. When I called out his name, he took off running. He was five years older, bigger, and taller, but no matter. I ran to his house and caught him trying to escape on his bike. I dragged him off. Before I threw a well-deserved punch, his mother burst through the front door.

"Leave my son alone, you bully."

I was taken aback. "I'm the bully? I'm a kid. He's in high school."

He saw an opening and ran to her side.

"And he just tried to kill me and my friend," I continued.

That sparked her curiosity. After I explained what happened, she realized the real bully had his arms wrapped around her.

In my freshman year at college, my professor, who was also chairman of the design department, flat out lied about what was covered on the midterm exam. Many had failed, many grumbled, but only I marched into his office and demanded he explain.

He smirked. "You must be prepared for everything."

Suspecting he would lie again on our remaining tests, I spread the word. True to form, he did not disappoint. I'm not sure about the other students, but I aced them all. When he announced his retirement during our last class of the year, I stared him in the eye from my front-row seat and began clapping. Not a polite round of applause, not one of celebration, but a thunderous salvo of good riddance. I hoped some, if not all, of the other forty-nine disgruntled students behind me would join in. Not one did, but I continued clapping, ignoring the fact that each clap drove another nail in the coffin of my design career before it had even begun. In the end, the chairman must have admired my chutzpah because I got an A minus for the course. I believe I deserved an A. Maybe I should have given him a standing ovation.

Sometimes I had fun dealing with less than honorable people. After a car accident in 1986, I began eighteen months of treatment with a chiropractor. Over that time, we got to know each other quite well, or so I thought. As I signed in for my last scheduled appointment, I asked the receptionist—the doctor's fiancée—to take down my new phone number.

"Why bother?" she said. "You're done."

My doctor echoed her response. I thought that was rude, and that both of their attitudes needed a major adjustment. But since picking a fight with your chiropractor prior to treatment could've been risky—"Do No Harm" may not apply here—I waited to exact my revenge.

After my final treatment, I got down on all fours and crawled out of his office and into the waiting room that was packed with nervous patients. I looked back and said, "Doc, I feel great. You're a miracle worker." His dirty look only spurred me on. So I crawled over to the receptionist, signed out, gave her a wink, and then continued on my hands and knees out the front door, down the hall to the elevator, never to return.

I have dealt with my share of conmen, liars, and rude people throughout my life, so with Tammy and the Tweedles, I was in familiar territory.

CHAPTER 26

There's a New Sheriff in Town

Mom: I should have my doggy blanket on me.

Me: He's down here at your feet.

Mom: But he should be up here so people can see him.

Me: Who?

Mom: All the wonderful neighbors.

W hen Mom whispered to me, "I don't like being alone. It's not pleasant," I realized those we hired to make sure she wasn't, often did. I did not seek an adversarial relationship with Tammy or the Tweedles. I only wanted to improve Mom's living conditions. But in their minds, I was the intruder, the homewrecker, the one who turned their world upside down. I guess I was.

All three tested my tolerance for laziness and my contempt for those who take advantage of people. I was raised in this house to be considerate of others, to appreciate hard work, and to take pride in a job well done. I saw little evidence of any of it from them. I tried my best to get along. I treaded carefully so as not to offend. When I chimed in with suggestions here and there, the Tweedles at least pretended to comply. Tammy made no effort. She only answered to Michael, whom I discovered she also ignored.

Yet he, my Brother Theresa, continued to defend this trio. I found his misplaced loyalty infuriating. The Porro recycling genes must have kicked in. He saw value in them when the rest of us did not. But, fortunately and unfortunately, I had the benefit of being on the front lines, watching them up close and in action over long periods of time. Without question, Mom had my loyalty.

Confident Michael would eventually see the light; I sucked it up, steeled my resolve, and pressed on. I stopped questioning why I constantly had to remind a "nurse's aide" to wear sanitary gloves, change the bedding daily, and for God's sake, treat Mom's horrendous bedsores. I stopped asking the Tweedles to clean up after themselves, to stop fighting me on everything, and, for God's sake, treat Mom with some respect.

But one can only take so much. When my dad reached his "that is all" moment with us kids, he reached for the wooden paddle he called "the Board of Education." Believe me, I was well-educated before I entered kindergarten. When I reached my "that is all" moment with Tammy, I instead asked to see her professional license. Several days later, she produced a xeroxed certificate emblazoned with a thirteen-year expiration date. New Jersey required renewal every twenty-four months, so I urged Michael once again to let me replace this phony with a legitimate aide. He admitted, perhaps for the first time, that he also had issues with Tammy, yet he still wavered. He did, however, agree to let me take over more of her shifts. I hoped she'd get the hint and leave on her own. She didn't.

Then the ticking time bomb I feared finally exploded when Michael forgot to leave Tammy her paycheck. She plowed through a snowstorm, trudged through the house, leaving puddles of melted snow in her wake, and screamed, "I want my fucking money!"

Nice. Finally, with a push from me—not quite a *she-goes-or-I-go ultimatum*, but pretty damn close—Michael showed Tammy and her bogus certification the door.

Putting up with Tammy a scant few hours a day was bad enough. Living under the same roof as the Tweedles for the unforeseeable future was sure to be a nightmare. The Tweedles, however, had a choice. They could move out at any time, but they had no intention of ever leaving our home.

I needed them gone, not only for Mom's well-being, but for my sanity. My preference— eviction—was ruled out for legal reasons, explained our attorney, who lived next door. We'd first met while I was standing on the front lawn peering through my mother's bedroom window one night. Since she fancied open curtains, I checked to see how visible her room was to the outside world. Being a vigilant neighbor, he approached. I introduced myself and told him what I was doing. He did the same. I then realized the only Peeping Toms we needed to worry about were the two of us.

With eviction off the table, it was time to move to plan B. We needed to set an end date and we needed it in writing. To get all parties on board, I suggested we make it the Tweedle toddler's last day of school in June, some six months away. With the added pressure from my other siblings, Michael reluctantly agreed to sign. The Tweedles, in no hurry to give up free living or free utilities, finally caved and added their signatures. I reintroduced the original list of duties they conveniently misplaced and, for the most part, ignored. Per our new agreement, the Tweedles would continue working until their departure, but that didn't last long. They gladly sat back while I—tired of beating a dead horse or, in this case, two—assumed more and more of their chores.

So, I committed to stay until the Tweedles moved out. After that, I wasn't sure. I hoped to get good people in place and then return to Los Angeles. But those six months with the Tweedles would surely test every inch of my moral fiber. My saving grace, my proverbial light at the end of the tunnel was that end date.

So, to survive I focused on that glorious, ever-brightening light, and to make sure no one forgot, especially *you know who*, I circled June 30, 2012 on the billboard-size calendar in the dining room for all to see.

CHAPTER 27

Our Champion of the Arts

*Mom: I've been thinking about blankets.
I'd like to have a different one.*

Me: What made you think of that?

Mom: Stamps.

Me: What kind of stamps, S&H?

*Mom: Yes. I filled the books and didn't know
what to get, so I'll get a blanket.*

I'd be hard-pressed to recall a dull moment growing up in Mom's world. It was always full of surprises; some welcome, some not so much. Like early morning boating and swimming lessons in the arctic waters of Ridgewood's Graydon Pool. I learned to appreciate those only after thawing out.

She always kept us busy. In between her shopping marathons and our various odd jobs, Mom took us on kid-friendly cultural excursions in New York City, thirty minutes away—or thirty hours, depending on traffic. We'd visit Radio City Music Hall to see the latest Disney film and behold the Rockettes' toes, in unison, pointing to the sky. Or we'd take in a Broadway play, hop on the ferry to the Statue of Liberty, or cruise around Manhattan on the Circle Line. At the 1964 World's Fair, I saw a "Jetson's-style" future and heard for the first time but unfortunately not the last, "It's A Small World After All." I have yet to get that damn song out of my head.

When I was ten years old, Mom took a gamble and hired a famous New York photographer to shoot test shots of all of us kids, hoping to ignite a modeling career or two, or six. After a full day of wardrobe and location changes, the only one the camera showed any affection for was Caryl, my blossoming teenage sister. But when only lingerie offers flooded in, she stuck with ballet. My only fond memory from that long day was a black-and-white photo of Louis Armstrong hanging in the bathroom. He sat on the toilet—the same toilet I sat on—holding a pack of cigarettes, while flashing his world-famous pearly whites.

Years later, after placing second in the Man of the Eighties contest in Columbus, Ohio—you made the finals if you owned a suit—I began my professional modeling career. My first gig, like Mom, was as a hand model. Or as my friends liked to say, "My first job was a hand job." That job led to more modeling jobs, which led to commercials, which led me to Hollywood. So, that early gamble was not a total loss for Mom.

She also shared with us her love for painting. Mom studied art before getting married. One of her oils hung in our living room, and I always thought it to be quite good. I'm sure having six kids played a part in halting her dream, but she never gave up supporting others. As a member of the Art Barn—a local gallery featuring artists from near and far—she'd take me to view the latest works and to help choose which painting to take home. Today, four of those paintings hang in my apartment in France.

However, we didn't need to leave the house for our fine arts fix. On Sunday nights, we huddled in the living room to watch the *Ed*

Sullivan Show. The Beatles, the plate twirlers, and that irresistible Italian mouse, Topo Gigio, were among our favorites. The dancers—ballet, modern, jazz, tap, flamenco—always got us on our feet for impromptu performances, much to Dad's chagrin. But when choreographer and local celebrity, Peter Gennaro, introduced his dancers, we sat right back down and focused. His creativity and talent always inspired us. Perhaps it was Peter who motivated Mom to sign all of us up for ballet lessons.

My dancing career started with a bang. Hollywood couldn't have written it any better. I was seven years old, visiting David and Caryl, who were performing with the Royal Danish Ballet at Lincoln Center in New York City.

A man stormed into the dressing room and shouted, "We need another kid." He locked eyes with me. "You, kid, wanna be in the show?"

I hesitated, not knowing what to say.

He quickly followed up with, "We'll pay you."

That was all I needed to hear. Now a professional, I'm off to my first makeup session and wardrobe fitting. In no time, I emerged dressed in a sweet swashbuckling costume with a frilly lace-up shirt, red sash, and a long plume in my cap that would have made Errol Flynn jealous. The only thing missing was a sword.

I soon joined my siblings atop a bridge towering above the stage filled with *other* professional dancers. However, we didn't do much dancing. Other than acting like we were having the best time—which we were—we, on cue, tossed paper flowers into the air and watched them cascade down onto the stage below, all for five dollars a show. I thought, *Why do they say a career in the arts is so difficult?*

Now, forty-seven years later, considering the last equity-waiver play I did in Los Angeles paid the same—five dollars a show—you can understand how *right* they were. In today's dollars, my showbiz debut turned out to be one of my best money-making years in the arts.

Though my Lincoln Center debut lasted only three shows, I was hooked. I started ballet lessons soon after and was thrilled by all the attention that came with being the only boy in my class. In fact, David and I were the only boys in the entire school. But what began with a bang ended with a thud three years later when my prima-donna attitude got me fired from *The Nutcracker*, two years running.

Irene Fokine's annual production of *The Nutcracker* drew a lot of talent from New York City. It was a big deal to be part of it, especially for a young dancer. In my first year, I played a boy at the opening party, the toy soldier who shot and killed the first mouse—I beat out a veteran for that role, no doubt due to all of my experience with mice at home. I also played a gnome who pulled the sleigh upon which the Prince and Clara traveled to all the magical lands. I had an issue with the gnome. First, I hated the green costume and curly-toed shoes with their glittery, bouncing balls. I couldn't let my friends see me dressed like this. Second, David played the Prince. I found no joy in pulling my brother around that stage and, worse, in *that* costume. Third, he sat in the sleigh next to Julie, who played Clara. I had a big crush on Julie. Every boy had a big crush on Julie, with her sparkling brown eyes, irresistible smile, and long wavy auburn hair. She was perfect.

On Sundays we did two shows: a matinee and an evening. In between, the cast changed into street clothes and grabbed a quick dinner.

During the first show, after killing the mouse, I got ready for dinner, except I wasn't finished. My gnome part remained. Ms. Fokine—our strict Russian teacher, choreographer, and disciplinarian—caught me before I escaped to the great outdoors.

"Get back here. You're not done."

I was in no mood to change clothes or get back into makeup. "Let my understudy go on," I said. Those words actually came out of my nine-year-old mouth.

She was not amused. "If you don't get in that costume, you're out of the show."

And that was that.

The next year, she cast me again as a gnome, and again, I left the show early. I wonder if my understudy became a big star like in the movies. If so, it's all thanks to me. Soon after, I quit ballet for good. Retired at ten years old.

But ballet gave me a lovely parting gift. During one of my last recitals, the lead dancer pirouetted off stage for a quick costume change, unaware I stood in the wings with an unobstructed view. There I caught my first glimpse of a woman's bare breasts. I stared in awe at the magnificent sight. Was this enough to keep me from quitting? No, but I've had an affinity for dancers and boobs ever since. Thank you, Barbara H. So, my ballet career, though short, was not a total loss for me.

CHAPTER 28

The Parade of Aides

Tweedle Dumb: Where are all the aides, huh?
Where are they?

Me: You're looking at 'em.

Job interviews can be nerve-racking for those on either side of the desk. As a designer, I had only a few interviews, and I nailed them all. As an actor, the chase never ends. You worry about the next job your entire career—for me, that worry lasted twenty-eight years. If fortunate, you audition often. You learn to read the room, the faces of the people asking questions, and especially the faces of those who don't. Knocking it out of the park can give you a euphoric sense of confidence. Causing the executive producer's jaw to drop can make you consider saying goodbye to Hollywood altogether. But I found the hiring side of the desk even more challenging. Even though I had little luck in finding good help for my past ventures, I hoped that was about to change.

We hired temporary aides to cover Tammy's shifts while we sought a permanent replacement. My intent was to remain as a part-time caregiver. I met with Anna, a reliable aide from the past, but after being left alone with Tweedle Dumb for just a moment, she disappeared, never to be seen again. I later found out that *someone* had scared her off with lies about me.

So, we placed an ad in search of a certified aide who had a valid driver's license, a good grasp of the English language, and who wasn't "batshit crazy" or a ticking time bomb, and whom Tweedle Dumb couldn't scare off. But be careful what you *don't* wish for. Several responses rolled in. I narrowed the list down to the three most promising candidates and scheduled interviews. If all went well, Michael and I would introduce them to Mom.

Candidate #1 Alice

Alice was a charming woman who had recently lost her long-time patient. Alice did fine during the interview and was thrilled to start as soon as possible, but when we introduced her to Mom, Alice took one look and melted into a puddle of tears. I quickly realized her emotional needs were more significant than Mom's practical ones. We passed.

Candidate #2 Lucia

Lucia, a sweet Central American woman arrived accompanied by six family members. Her oldest daughter did most of the talking. Lucia answered every question with, "I ruv yu mudda," which I soon realized was all the English she knew. So, I asked her daughter to translate for her "mudda."

"What happens if there's an emergency and Lucia needs to call the hospital?"

The daughter fell silent. I bristled.

Sensing my concern, Lucia smiled her best smile and said the most unhelpful words in such a situation, "I ruv yu mudda."

We did too. So, we passed.

Candidate #3 Sonia

Sonia, a Jamaican nurse, arrived in her uniform—a plus. A silent yet intimidating husband accompanied her, not such a plus. She spoke English and had a valid driver's license—plus, plus. Sonia worked at a local hospital, needed the extra income, and Mom approved—the pluses won. She agreed to a trial period of two weeks at $15 an hour. During the interview, Sonia jokingly called Michael the Devil and me the Devil's advocate. It struck us as funny at first. We never gave it much thought until she kept repeating it. And like a dog with a tasty bone, she never let it go.

On her first day, I came home to find Mom and Sonia sitting at the kitchen table.

Sonia: I'm worth more than $15 an hour.

Me: (taken aback) You haven't even finished one day. We agreed to $15 an hour for two weeks. We'll discuss a raise after.

Sonia: Okay, but I'm overqualified at $15 an hour.

Me: Duly noted.

Day two and every day after, as soon as I set foot in the kitchen, Sonia hit me with the same complaint: "I'm worth more than $15 an hour." But since Mom liked her, I bit my tongue and prayed for the strength to endure what could now be called the "Jamaican Torture Test." Michael got his chance to experience my joy when he came one Tuesday evening. He never returned.

Out of desperation, I begged Sonia. "Please stop. Honor the deal you agreed to."

She said she feared we would not pay her.

"Why would you think that?"

"Because you are the Devil's advocate," she barked.

Okay, this was no longer funny. With no more tongue left to bite, I gritted my teeth and focused on that couldn't-arrive-soon-enough last day of my Jamaican hell.

When that day finally came, I returned home to find Mom and Sonia in the living room. She got in one last grumble about the low wages before announcing, "I'm done with this job."

Unable to contain my sense of relief, I said, "Damn right, you are." But goodbyes are never easy.

Michael, who handled all of Mom's finances, and who also liked to spring the occasional surprise, had yet another one for me. "It's snowing. I'm not coming to pay Sonia." Then added casually, "Anyway, I'm out of checks." His solution? "Have Mom sign one."

I didn't know the last time Mom had signed anything. She had gorgeous handwriting, and her signature was fine art, but after her stroke in 1993, I feared I'd never see it again. Mom being Mom, had fully recovered, as did her penmanship, but that was nineteen years ago. Of the six Porro siblings, only Laurel's hand came close. However, Laurel lived in sunny California, and forgery was not an option, at least one I wasn't willing to entertain . . . yet.

The end of my nightmare all depended on finding a checkbook, if one still existed in this house, and a signature, if Mom could still manage one. I explained to Sonia the predicament the Devil, her name for Michael—which fit at that moment—had put us in. Then I went in search of Mom's checkbook. *Eureka.* When I returned with it, a pen and a pad, Sonia seethed.

Sonia: All my suspicions about the Devil and his advocate are coming true. You were going to rip me off the whole time.

Me: Why would you think that?

Sonia: Because you are the Devil's advocate!

Me: Everything will be fine. Mom will sign your check.

(I handed Mom the pen and pad.)

Me: Mom, practice your signature.

Sonia: *(patting Mom's hand)* You are a sweet old lady, Gen. I love you. (To me) But you're an asshole.

(Ignoring her, I checked on Mom. After a few attempts of signing her name, she was dead asleep.)

Sonia: That old lady can't sign a check.

Me: *(upbeat)* Yes, she can. She has beautiful handwriting.

(I nudged Mom awake.)

Me: Mom, can you please sign your name?

With both sets of eyes on her, Mom scribbled a G and part of an E before drifting off again.

Sonia: *(erupting)* She can't sign it. Look at her. I knew you two would rip me off. You're a fucking asshole.

(Mom woke up. Sonia grabbed Mom's hand.)

Sonia: But, Gen, I love you.

(I begged Mom to try again, but the pen trailed off the page as her head fell. I woke her and desperately urged her to keep trying.)

Sonia: I'm Black. I'll be arrested trying to cash that check. I'm very disappointed. You scammed me. You think I'm stupid? This is my last day.

Me: *(an attempt at levity)* But I didn't get to review you yet. Is now a good time?

Sonia: I'm not here for the money, but I want my $400.

Me: I can go to an ATM and get $300. You can come back for the balance.

Sonia: *(exploding)* I'm not getting in a car with you!

Me: Okay, you're angry. I'd like you to leave.

Sonia: *(raising her voice to new heights)* I am not angry! And I am not leaving without my money!

Me: Please leave this house now because you do not want to see me angry.

Sonia: What are you going to do?

Me: *(calm but dead serious)* You do not want to see me angry.

Sonia: I'm going to call the police and have you arrested.

Me: Go ahead, call. Who do you think they'll arrest?

Sonia checked her watch. It was 8:00 p.m.

Sonia: I have to get your mother ready.

Me: You will not touch my mother again. Please leave.

(Eavesdropping on the entire tête-à-tête, Tweedle Dee bounded down the steps, gasping for air.)

Tweedle Dee: I have cash. I can pay you.

(I looked at her in disbelief.)

I had recently discovered the Tweedles charged $340 in long-distance calls to my mother's account and refused to pay it back. And they had that much cash sitting around? Surprised and yet relieved, I saw it as the only way to end my current nightmare.

(Tweedle Dee handed me $400.)

Me: Does that work for you, Sonia?

Sonia: Yes, but you are still the Devil's advocate.

Me: *(handing her the cash)* Fine. Please go.

Sonia: And your brother is the Devil.

Me: Go.

Sonia: I'm going.

She stormed out and ranted all the way to her car. So much for avoiding a batshit-crazy ticking time bomb. After locking and bolting the front door, I thanked Tweedle Dee for coming to my rescue. Although tempted to put that cash toward their phone bill, I decided *one* issue a night was enough. I said goodnight with a promise to reimburse her the next day.

Mom and I weathered the Jamaican Torture Test relatively unscathed. After putting her to bed, I settled down in the living room and stared at her scribbles on the practice pad. And just like Sonia, Mom's beautiful John Hancock was gone forever.

CHAPTER 29

Not Another Fire, Please

*Me: How is it that you find the need
to fight me on everything?*

Tweedle Dumb: I do not.

Me: Yes, you do.

Tweedle Dumb: I do not.

Me: You're doing it right now.

Tweedle Dumb: That's your opinion.

Me: It's not my opinion. It's a fact.

Tweedle Dumb: Well, I don't agree with it.

Once their departure date was set, the Tweedles stayed pretty much out of sight. *Thank God for small favors.* They only came downstairs to cook their meals, but always scurried back up to eat them. Tweedle

Dumb had been careless about many things, but when it came to fire, she seemed to throw all caution to the wind. She counted on luck, dumb luck as it turned out. After intervening in a couple of close calls, I considered it a miracle that another fire hadn't engulfed 247 Emmett while they were in charge.

The first time was when I found an empty yet blazing-hot toaster oven heating the entire kitchen, and with no one in sight. I turned it off and moved it a safe distance from the wall while it cooled along with my nerves. At this point in our cohabitation, besides avoiding me at all costs, Tweedle Dumb demanded we only communicate in writing. Being more critical than them leaving the doors open or the lights on, I asked the quieter, less-combative Tweedle Dee to tell her mother to please turn the toaster oven off before leaving the kitchen. As usual, Tweedle Dee took offense and marched upstairs to deliver my message. Judging by the sudden thunder rolling down the steps, it was not well received.

Tweedle Dumb had never accepted any responsibility for any of the problems she was responsible for. Why would I think she'd start now? So, I braced for yet another battle. She stormed into the kitchen and slammed a stack of mail on top of the gas stove with its robust pilot light glowing below. I thought placing flammables near an open flame was no way to start the argument we were about to have.

She fired away at full volume, "I know how to use a toaster oven. I've owned twenty-three houses."

"And how many of those have you burned down?" I couldn't resist asking.

She sneered, insisting the toaster oven automatically shut off.

"Yes, if you set it for timed cooking. Otherwise, it stays on forever. Like it did today," I said.

She refused to accept that simple fact and continued to defend herself for several more minutes. Hoping to end yet another circular argument, I offered to demonstrate toaster oven basics.

"I'll just pull the plug from now on," she countered before stomping out in a huff.

Even better, I thought.

I'd caught another near miss the previous winter when I returned to a dark house while everyone slept, except for the fireplace shooting glowing embers onto the wood floor. *Someone,* mum's the word, had left the protective screen and glass doors wide open before retiring upstairs. When I left a note, per her wishes, Tweedle Dumb mulled it over for a day or two, then logged her defense in writing, once again freeing herself of all responsibility and closed with:

"I don't want you to worry. I have owned twenty-three houses. I know what I'm doing, okay?"

Her long past tiresome claim prompted my snarky response. "Then you should have no trouble finding number twenty-four. It ain't this one."

The Porros tend to be sensitive about house fires. For us, the most significant event in July 1969 was not the one-small-step-for-man moon landing, but a five-alarmer that destroyed the second story of our house.

Thankfully, no one was hurt. However, we lost many irreplaceable items, including collections of near-priceless vintage baseball cards and comic books, our stockpile of Wiffle balls (in two sizes, no less), and Aurora Plastics classic models of Frankenstein's monster, the Mummy, the Phantom of the Opera, Dr. Jekyll as Mr. Hyde, Dracula, and my favorite, John F. Kennedy from the Great American Presidents series. JFK sat in his rocking chair in the Oval Office. He wore my preferred color of socks: white. I took a lot of ribbing from my big brothers about my lack of presidential fashion sense, but if anyone other than me could rock white socks, it was JFK.

The fire also destroyed my acting debut in Michael J. Porro's Super 8 epic film, *Adam in the Garden of Eden*. At eight years old, I starred as Adam. I'd entered the set—our vestibule packed with every Eden-like plant in the house—buck naked except for a well-placed but not well-secured fig leaf. On the first take, my nerves got the best of me. The leaf tumbled and took my Hollywood dreams with it. Instead of going on with the show, I'd quit the business in shame. But we all know how Hollywood loves a comeback. Twenty-one years later, I made my triumphant return. As a proud new member of the Screen Actors Guild, I landed my first role on television as Assistant District Attorney Simmons on the Emmy-Award-winning series, *Hill Street Blues*. And many more acting jobs followed.

On the day of the fire, I was grounded, but I snuck out via my usual escape route, hanging out the second-story window, grabbing hold of the gutter, shinnying across to the porch roof, then sliding down the gutter pipe to freedom.

Earlier in the spring, my escape to the porch roof led to another kind of freedom. Sue, my first official girlfriend and my first kiss, was a dark-haired beauty with braces to whom I'd professed my initial attraction by launching her shoes high into a pine tree where they still might be. Mating rituals were different back then. ID bracelets meant you were "Going Steady. When her father discovered Sue with mine, he demanded she return it. "Fifth graders are too young to go steady, and especially with a long-haired boy."

For the record, my hair barely touched my ears. But per her father's wishes, Sue came to my house, stood below my bedroom window, and called out my name. Sensing the inevitable, I shinnied across to the porch roof, but no further.

"To make the breakup official, you must throw my bracelet and I must catch it," I insisted. I dropped the first three attempts on purpose before ending her frustration and officially beginning my heartbreak on the fourth. Single again at eleven. Reflecting on my first girlfriend experience, I hedged my bets by sealing the deal with a cheap 007 ID bracelet instead of the expensive engraved one my parents had given me. I had commitment issues even back then. Fittingly, both bracelets perished in the fire.

While flames engulfed 247 Emmett Place, I hung out a mile away at Veteran's Field. Later that afternoon, a friend of my brother Michael spotted me and yelled, "Your house is on fire."

I didn't believe him. "Oh yeah, which one?"

"Third from the end."

I laughed. "That's our horrible neighbor's house. Good for them."

He approached and looked me straight in the eye. "I know your house. It's on fire. I'll drive you." He seemed sure, so I went.

Fire trucks, big and small, lined our street. A crowd jostled for an unobstructed view in front of my house. Thick fire hoses snaked through the front door. A team of firefighters stood on the roof, battling the flames below. Was my family safe? I knew my father was at baseball practice, and Mom and Deecy were at Sunday Mass. But Michael, David, and Caryl were home when I'd snuck out. I scanned the crowd and found them. Everyone was okay. Hours later, as the firefighters packed up their gear, our cat, Casper, staggered out of the front door, in shock but unharmed, with most of his fur still white. Our fire made the front page of the *Ridgewood News* that week. And forty-three years later, though most of the second floor was rebuilt, a few scars, chars, and a burned-wood smell remained throughout the attic spaces. I spent a lot of my youth in those spaces. Since then, I always erred on the side of caution because of that pungent smell.

I suspected Mom had witnessed previous incidents by the Tweedles since she never again enjoyed a cozy fire on a cold winter night, even while I tended it. We had been lucky so far. But if that luck ran out and I wasn't home, I could only imagine how far down my mother would have landed on the Tweedles' priority list.

CHAPTER 30

Single, Fifty-Five, and Living with My Mother

Who said you can't go home again? —Me

After the parade of aides failed to deliver a winner, I decided to take over all of my mother's care on a full-time basis. That meant moving back into my childhood home, no longer as a visitor but as a resident. A home I hadn't lived in since I'd left for college. A home not only with my mother but with three lovely roommates and their menagerie of pets. I hadn't lived with roommates in over twenty-six years, or with pets in over thirty-five (I'm allergic to most pets. Most roommates too). Safe to say this wasn't my original plan, if there had ever been one. I initially came to rescue my mom and to take some of the burden off Michael's shoulders, but circumstances changed. It was time to step up, step up big time.

To seal the deal, I shipped my Prius, my guitar, and the rest of my clothes from the dry heat of Los Angeles summers to the high humidity of New Jersey's. Since sleeping in the living room offered no privacy, I cleared out the back bedroom and bought a new bed, a comfortable one. The decades-old hide-a-backbreaker no longer cut it, not that it ever did. And I settled into my new reality as best as I could.

When introducing myself to a neighbor—an attractive psychiatrist from Lithuania—I joked, "I'm single, fifty-five, and I live with my mother. You're going to want me on your couch." She laughed and we became fast friends.

Okay, I realize at first blush "living with your mother" doesn't bode well for anyone over eighteen, let alone a man in his fifties. I didn't really care how it looked to others. I was on a mission. But if I did care, hopefully by the end of this story I'd emerge smelling like a rose. If not, an attractive psychiatrist from Lithuania who lives across the street is going to hear all about it.

CHAPTER 31

The UPC Label Mystery

Who threw out those cheese labels? —Mom

Mom's obsession with Universal Product Codes began years ago when she discovered if she collected enough and mailed them in—along with a substantial check—a beautiful collector's item awaited at the end of the UPC rainbow. That was all she needed to hear. Whenever we opened a bag, a box, a bottle, a jar, or a can in our house, we always heard, "Save the label."

Hoarding UPCs just gave her another excuse to shop. She bought things she didn't need, for labels no one else saved, to get junk no one else wanted. The only people who collected these "precious" items were suckers like Mom, who, unfortunately, were in ample supply. In every nook and cranny of our house, a *collectible* could be found. Things like the Black Tower wine bottle telephone, the Campbell's limited-edition ceramic soup can, and the Jolly Green Giant Little Green Sprout alarm clock.

In 1993, during our fourth family reunion in the quaint, quiet town of Holland on the shore of the Great Lakes State, Mom shattered all tranquility when she shared her UPC obsession with everybody in, on, or near Lake Michigan.

My two brothers and I, along with our teenage nephew, Abe, were battling for the beach croquet championship fifty yards away when we first heard the rumblings deep inside our vacation house.

"Did you throw those labels out? Did you? I brought that cheese all the way from New Jersey."

Her voice grew louder as she marched from room to room, rummaging through trash can after trash can, tearing into any and all suspects who were unfortunate enough to be in her path.

"I need those labels. Who threw them out?"

We grew up with her, so this odd behavior, although a bit overboard, was amusing rather than shocking. But it was just the opposite for my nephew. Still, he felt relatively safe fifty yards away in the deep sand with Lake Michigan as an escape route. But after watching that *crazed thing* possessing his grandmother's body emerge from the house, dig through every community garbage bin, and then zero in on the four of us, all bets were off.

As she made a beeline through the sand, her face raging red, her weaponized "Take No Prisoners" finger waving at us Porro boys, Abe inched toward the water.

"Did one of *you* throw out my cheese labels?"

But nobody interrupts beach croquet, the championship game no less, not even our mother. I don't remember who started it, but as soon as she closed in and pointed that loaded finger, one of us hit the sand as if being shot. And the others followed. Again and again, she pointed. Again and again, we fell. We then pretended to struggle to our feet, only to take another dive as soon as *that* finger found us. We continued this charade until she threw her hands up in frustration and trudged back to the house. There, she focused her rage on the next victim, Michael's wife, but Mom met her match with Diane. We listened to the fireworks from a safe distance away in the deep sand, with Lake Michigan as our escape route.

Later, a much-relieved Abe said that watching his grandmother attack three grown men was the funniest thing he'd ever seen. That was our goal. We didn't want Mom's first grandchild to fear her or her quirks.

What motivated Mom's collector-item passion that day remains a mystery, but I can guarantee that Abe never touched another one of her UPC labels ever again.

CHAPTER 32

I Am My Mother's Son

Mom: What have they got to eat?
Me: I'm the "they."
Mom: Well, what have you got?

J ust like that, as soon as I took over, reality hit. My mother made her priorities as clear as a dinner bell.
"I'm hungry. Feed me."
It didn't matter who fed her. Only what and when. And she could be mean about it after depending on others for so long, some of whom couldn't have cared less. But I did care. My goal was to restore what had been whittled away over the past four and a half years: her dignity. But first, I had to feed her.
Other than her long red nails, she had little

else to feel good about. She wore no makeup, no lipstick, and her long hair was often coiled in a lifeless bun. Her nightshirts, which doubled as day shirts, were old, drab, and tattered. Her socks were slippery and dangerous.

The first order of business was a new wardrobe, including, for safety reasons, non-slip socks. That meant shopping. Nothing would please her more or please me less. But since this was to be a surprise, I kept quiet, made an excuse, and snuck out to the mall on my own. A middle-aged man shopping for nightgowns for his ninety-year-old mother shouldn't be too uncomfortable, right?

Wrong. Not only was it uncomfortable as hell, but it was also disappointing. After rummaging through the racks in several stores and dealing with stares from young salesgirls and dirty old women, I found the same drab nightshirts that doubled as day shirts like the ones Mom already owned, only newer and not yet tattered. Other than identifying an untapped fashion niche (someone should get on that), I struck out.

But as my mother's son, determined to fulfill not only a want but a need, and living in the twenty-first century, I went shopping online. I looked up night dresses, nightshirts, and nightgowns for seniors. Hoping to find something bright, comfortable, age appropriate, and functional, as in easy-on-easy-off, I came up empty. (I'm serious, someone needs to address that gold mine of a market niche). So I deleted "age appropriate" and tried again.

Bingo. An abundance of options filled the computer screen. My next problem: choosing. After careful consideration, I ordered several stretchy cotton nightdresses in colors that complemented Mom's complexion: pink, blue, and one—dare I say it—in sexy black. All with long sleeves for storing her well-worn tissues and on the short side to show off her still-shapely legs. The new gowns were a hit. She loved them, she looked good in them, and she received several compliments.

To keep my errand running to a minimum, I shopped more and more online. I bought adult diapers, Pro-Stat, sanitary gloves, and a suitable sippy cup. Sippy cups were most challenging due to Mom's limited flexibility and sucking capacity, which I imagine most seniors lack (another market niche that needs attention). She tried several bright-colored, hard-to-grasp, alien-like cups with short nipple spouts. All were nearly impossible to draw out even a drop. My search contin-ued until I found a Genevieve-friendly design: simple, easy to hold, and with a replaceable bendable straw. But I quickly learned a critical new parent lesson when her never-out-of-sight sippy cup went out of sight. Always have a backup! So, back online I went, and two new sippy cups arrived a week later. One day I would get this parenting thing down.

For peace of mind, I ordered a video baby monitor with night vision to keep tabs on her. Though no threat to leave her bed, I worried she might need something when I was out of earshot. Like me, Mom was a night owl. She spent many waking hours sleeping, so she had energy to burn at night. She fidgeted, appeared to see things, and talked to them. I couldn't see what she saw or make out what she said, but I couldn't take my eyes off my iPhone. I watched like an obsessed reality show fan who had nothing better to do, like sleep. Even though some evenings were better than most shows on television, binge-watching Mom all night caused me more anxiety than if I'd just stayed in her room.

CHAPTER 33

The Battle of the Dutch Door

Shut the door! —Mom

The Dutch door. Common in the Netherlands in the seventeenth century, Dutch settlers brought their split door to the United States, where it first appeared in rural houses in New York and New Jersey. It had been originally designed as an exterior door to keep children in and animals out while allowing air and light to come and go. My dad didn't have any Dutch in his blood, but he liked the Dutch door concept. His homemade interior Dutch door let air and light come and go but kept children and pets out of the kitchen until we wiped our feet and cleaned our paws.

Whenever we flew out the side door or down the basement steps and forgot to close the top and bottom, Mom's "Shut the door!" always rang out to remind us. Nowadays, she liked the top open for the sunshine and fresh air, but Tweedle Dumb never obliged.

"Why do you keep closing the door?" I asked.

"There's poison in the basement," she claimed. "Blackie ate it once, convulsed, and threw up."

"Well, if that's true, cats are smart. I'm sure he won't do that again," I said. "Mom likes the door open while she eats. You can keep Blackie upstairs during that time."

She, of course, objected, and the Battle of the Dutch Door began. Whenever I stepped out of the kitchen, Tweedle Dumb stepped in and slammed the door shut while Mom, helpless in her wheelchair, could only watch. I'd go back and open it. This nonsense continued back and forth until I threatened to remove the door altogether.

"How happy we'd be if you were as attentive to my mother as you are to your cat," I added.

Tweedle Dumb responded with her rarest of gifts: silence.

After that, the top remained open at mealtime. The Battle of the Dutch Door was over, or so I thought. Occasionally, I'd also leave the bottom ajar. This reignited the old tug-of-war with Mom. Though I may have forgotten her "Shut the door" refrain from my childhood, she had not. As I wheeled her into the kitchen, Mom would always check the door. If it was open, she'd reach out and close it in one smooth move as we rounded the table, and without saying a word. Thus, a new yet most welcome Battle of the Dutch Door began. I got such a kick out of it that I left the bottom open on purpose every day.

At the time, I had no idea how vital a role that our battle would play in our journey. My simple action: leaving the bottom open, created an entertaining yet telling reaction on Mom's part: closing it. This signaled to me that all was well. But when she stopped, I'd know our battle was over, and that the end was near.

CHAPTER 34

Give Me a Break

I love my job, I love my job, I love my job . . .
—My mantra

Twenty-four-seven caregiving, especially for a loved one, is both physically and emotionally draining. Experts say, "Breaks are critical to avoid your own significant health problems." Even though Deecy and I took daily walks while on death watch back in February, I now resisted breaks. I thought I could handle it. In 1995, I dealt with the stress and strain—albeit for only sixteen days—of trekking through Italy with little knowledge of the language while caring for my eighty-year-old father who was battling heart disease. I didn't know if he'd make it back home safe and sound, let alone alive. But he survived.

I was in familiar territory with Mom. I was

at home, I knew the language, and she was in better shape. So, what's the big deal?

"What's the big deal"? Didn't Evel Knievel say something like that before launching himself into instead of over the Snake River Canyon?

I had been running my snack-food business since 1998. During the darkest and most stressful moments—of which there were many—I often relied on my mantra. It also turned out to be quite useful in my new life as Mom's caregiver. On the cusp of losing all hope, I didn't go negative, I went positive. And if I said "I love my job" over and over again, I just might believe it. If not, on to wine. Preferably red, and plenty of it.

We hadn't been out much since I'd moved back in December 2011. I thought a breath of fresh air would do us both some good. So, as Mom liked to say, we went "gallivanting." We Jersey-Shored it for Caryl's royal spa treatment. We drove to Long Island to see Aunt Claire, the last of Dad's siblings—which turned out to be their last visit.

Closer to home, we tracked down old favorites only to discover time had erased many of them. Tice's and Van Riper's Farms had been replaced by a strip mall. These were the go-to places in the fall for fresh apple cider and red candy apples, and the best place to lose yourself in an intoxicating cloud of cinnamon. Fishel's Bakery, the home of melt-in-your-mouth cream donuts and ice-cream cakes, no longer existed. Mama Rosa's pizza—the pizza by which I measure all others—vanished. T&W Ice Cream, who made the tastiest chocolate chip mint—gone. No sign of the Dairy Queen where David and I had worked at in high school, or Thom McAn shoes, who'd made the best penny loafers for competitive sliding on smooth winter ice. The delicatessen that replaced Pat's now overcharged unsuspecting customers for every sandwich and took exception when I called them out. You never had to count your change with Pat.

We attended Easter Mass at Our Lady of Mount Carmel, where even at church, Porsches, Mercedes, and Jaguars stole the scarce "handicap parking" spaces. This confirmed my belief that the disabled only drive the swankiest cars. I don't believe the lack of morals qualifies as a disability, but perhaps *these* car owners do. Though Mom couldn't remember her last

Mass, I would think a lack of mobility and near-death qualified as valid excuses for any lapse in the eyes of the Church. So, heaven for her, and not the morally disabled, should still be in the cards. We also stopped by Valleau cemetery to say hi to Dad. It had been fifteen years since we laid him to rest, and I was sure at least a couple of years since Mom's last hello. Her lack of mobility and near-death qualified here too.

She sat stern and silent for a few minutes. Then she whispered, "I miss ya."

Once again, I was reduced to tears.

Although I enjoyed these jaunts with Mom, I had yet to take a proper day or night off for myself. Stress could creep up on me, especially when lack of sleep was the new norm.

One night, after having a difficult time, I yelled, "If you really don't want to be here anymore, why don't you go ahead and die?"

I regretted those words as soon as they passed my lips.

A few weeks later, stress got the best of me again and culminated in a flash of rage. Mom descended into one of her dark moods and refused to eat her dinner.

"Fine," I said.

Okay, I need to clarify something. In my family, the word "fine" doesn't necessarily mean "good," "satisfactory," or "very well." It could be, and at times was, an undeniable "fuck you." If Deecy or I ever ended an argument with "fine," the other quickly asked, "What kind of 'fine' are we talking about?"

In this instance with Mom, it was the undeniable kind.

After my "Fine," I grabbed her salad bowl and smashed it. A large piece ricocheted and hit the stove's tempered glass door, shattering then scattering what seemed like millions of tiny sizzling diamonds across the entire kitchen floor.

"Are you okay?" I asked, panicked.

Mom nodded, and upon inspection, she was unharmed. Fortunately, my body had shielded her from the flying glass. The only damage was to the oven door, the bowl, the salad, and perhaps my ego.

I ordered new glass, and when I was installing it, I asked Mom, "Do you remember what happened here?"

She flashed a sly smile. "I have no idea."

I took that as a sign of forgiveness, one of her best virtues.

But *that* outburst did it for me. I finally gave in and yielded to the experts. I scheduled dinner and a movie with an old friend in New York City. After Mom ate, I sat her in the red reclining chair—with an extra bed pad beneath her just in case—to watch *Wheel of Fortune* and *Jeopardy*. David dropped by for a rare before midnight visit, and the Tweedles were home. I believed I had a support team in place when I left for my much-needed escape.

When I returned, I found Mom alone in the dark, in the reclining chair where I had left her several hours ago. But now she was sitting in a cold, wet diaper on top of a urine-soaked bed pad while the Tweedles slept upstairs, snug, and warm in their dry beds. Once again, they never failed to disappoint.

I didn't take any more breaks until they moved out. But that night, after cleaning Mom up and putting her to bed, I opened a bottle of red and repeated to myself, "I love my job, I love my job, I love my job . . ."

CHAPTER 35

Reality Will Be Unkind to You

Tweedle Dumb: You need therapy.
You have a problem.

Me: I do, and I'm looking at it.

Wired to blame others, engage in circular arguments, and wallow in lies, Tweedle Dumb missed her calling: a career in politics. The truth didn't come easy for her, nor did reality. But as we approached the end of their stay, the floodgates finally burst open, and it was delicious.

"We were deceived from the very beginning. Your mother is crazy, and she's depressed, but we already moved here, so we were stuck with no place to go."

I struggled to make sense of this. "And yet you stayed for four years?"

"Four and a half this summer," she corrected.

This didn't help her argument. I've always liked this quote, "'Tis better to be thought a fool than open one's mouth and remove all doubt." Tweedle Dumb opened her mouth far too often, and sometimes only long enough to exchange feet.

Both Tweedles relished their new roles as squatters. Not only did they stop doing most of their chores, they also did everything in their power to make my life miserable up until their very last minute of their very last day. I must admit, I returned the favor, although with a bit more finesse.

It was a mistake to give them six months' notice. It still confounds me why I even suggested it. I guess I had a little of my Brother Teresa in me too. We lost those precious months of Mom's happiness by having them remain in our house. And for that, I may never forgive myself.

When *Freedom Day* finally arrived and the Tweedles' four years—forgive me—four and a half years came to a close, I had so much I wanted to say to Tweedle Dumb, but I left it at, "Reality will be unkind to you."

Upon their departure, as expected, the Tweedles left a mess, left the lights on, and left their unpaid $340 long-distance phone bill. But they were gone. No more roommates. No more unwanted pets. No more surprises. Our house was once again our home sweet home with just Mom and me.

CHAPTER 36

You Don't See Them?

(Mom stares intensely at the ceiling)

Mom: Look at the chocolate coats.

Me: The what?

Mom: The kids with chocolate coats.

Me: Made of chocolate?

Mom: No silly, chocolate color. They're on the ceiling.

Me: Who's being silly?

I don't know why, but I checked on Mom earlier than usual. Most mornings she'd be sound asleep. Occasionally, she'd be up and calling for hot tea or cold juice. She had been a coffee drinker when she was younger but had lost the taste for it during her pregnancy with yours truly. Ever since, hot tea, skim milk, no sugar became her beverage of choice. Feeling partially responsible for the hit taken by the coffee market, I French-pressed my fair share of ground arabica beans to make up for it.

But on this particular morning, she surprised me. She was wide awake, unusually chipper, and not at all thirsty. Her hazel eyes twinkled as she gazed out the bedroom window. These days, any activity she saw out there provided more thrills than anything on television. Sometimes it was Dr. Irma, draped in her white lab coat, returning home from a long day at the Pines Psychiatric Hospital. Sometimes it was Betty, a retired nurse, clad in one of her authentic Scottish Highlands pure-wool kilts, walking Scottie, her Welsh Corgi, his belly hovering just above the sidewalk. Sometimes it was a brown cottontail rabbit hopping across the front lawn after gorging on Mom's daisies. But whatever she had seen that day was different.

Me: What's out there, Momma?

Mom: You don't see them?

She pointed to the window. I looked but saw nothing but a crumbling sidewalk crying for rejuvenation.

Me: See who?

Mom: The children. Heavens to Betsy, look at
    all of them walking by.
    She smiled and waved. I checked again. I still
    saw nothing.
Mom: With balloons. Oh, there's another with
    flowers. Lots of flowers have gone by, too.
Me: Recognize anyone?
Mom: I'm sure I do. Some of them. There's a
    yellow balloon.
Me: Any relatives?
Mom: *(teasing)* Maybe.
Me: Any inviting you to join them?
    She answered only with a sly grin.
Me: *(pressing)* Mom?
Mom: *(sneering)* No.
Me: Good.
Mom: You don't see them?
Me: No, sorry.
Mom: If you go out on the sidewalk, you will.
Me: Maybe later. Ready for breakfast?
Mom: In a minute.
Me: Okay, call me when you are.
Mom: There's a girl with daisies. I love
    daisies.
Me: I know, Momma. Enjoy the parade.

On my way out, my eyes landed on the old black-and-white photo hanging on the front wall. In it, eight-year-old Genevieve, dressed in a frilly white dress, white lace socks, and patent-leather shoes, sits on a bench holding a posy of daisies. The thought of how perfect this little girl would fit right in with Mom's parade made me chuckle.

As a young teen, my grandmother shared with me disturbing stories of her neighbor trashing her lawn and denting her car. Angry and eager to confront the SOB, I couldn't believe no one wanted to join me. My aunt Flo cooled me off with the truth. They called it dementia back then. Fortunately, Grandma's delusions lightened up after she moved into a nursing home. When Dad visited, if she didn't mistake him for her husband, she'd say things like, "You're lucky to catch me. I don't usually work on Tuesdays."

Mom had many visions early in our journey. Most were light, some dark, and others damn entertaining. But this parade of children was the first she'd described in such detail. And though she would see them march down Emmett Place many times after, I was relieved that none of the children beckoned her to join them, at least not on that day.

CHAPTER 37

If You Rebuild It, They Will Return

Mom: I'm sad.

Me: How can you be sad? You have
your health and a house
that's getting more and more beautiful
each day.

Mom: Who's paying for all that?

Me: You are. So, cheer up. You may have to
go back to work.

247 Emmett Place was built in the 1930s, back when two-by-fours actually measured two by four. Our family created many fond and some not-so-fond memories over our sixty-plus years there, but our house

had been abused and neglected for too many years. It needed not just minor repairs but a major renovation. I had a new project: return some dignity to our home. I hoped this would help lift Mom's spirits as well as mine, and since she slept many hours of the day, I had the time to take it on.

I had acquired many design and construction skills over the years and honed them in 2003 while building the factory for my snack-food company in Los Angeles. My erratic contractor had given me constant hell for a year and a half, greeting me every day with comments like, "You swing a hammer like a chick," and, "You want to fuck up your wrenches, keep using them like that." But I was on a mission at that time, so I put up with his abuse while soaking up all of his knowledge. Sadly, our master-bitch relationship hit a bump midway to completion when he chose to make his point with a pipe rather than words. The ensuing restraining order sealed his fate. I took my newfound skills, finished the project on my own, and turned that abandoned warehouse into an impressive organic food processing facility. Only when the psychological scars fully healed could I say that my eighteen months of misery was worth it. In the meantime, I carried my new skills with me to several projects since, so going through that hell had its benefits.

I began with the disaster in the basement while *you know who* still dwelled on the second floor. Clearing their junk, tearing down water-damaged paneling, and beating the crap out of termite-infested studs provided much-needed stress relief from *you know who*. I found it satisfying, exhilarating, and calming all at the same time.

Next, their domain. My dad had updated the upstairs bathroom after the fire in 1969. It featured a boy's side with a sink, a toilet, and a shower; and a girl's side with two sinks, a toilet, and a bathtub. A wall with a built-in radiator, open on both sides, separated the two rooms. This invited peeking, which also invited a good scolding if one got caught while Laurel soaked in the tub. I'm not saying who got caught spying. Mum's the word.

The combination of materials before and after the fire made dismantling a challenge. The sheer weight of the original cast-iron tub and concrete shower pan made it impossible to remove without jackhammering them into manageable pieces. The floor was a four-layer sandwich: tiles from 1969 covered linoleum and quarter-inch plywood from the 1950s, which was nailed to three-quarter-inch plywood from the 1930s. It took forever to tear up the quarter-inch plywood held down by hundreds of nails randomly distributed over one hundred square feet of floor. The largest piece measured two-by-two inches. My father led a remarkably frugal life—he wore shoes older than me—yet he spared no expense on the nails securing that floor. I never cursed him until that day.

Once stripped down to the rafters, I envisioned an open-plan bathroom with one toilet, a two-sink vanity, a large bathtub, a frameless glass shower, recessed lights, and a radiant-heated floor, which would be luxurious on cold winter mornings.

The rebuilding phase required daily trips to the Home Depot, which was thankfully close by. As a special treat for Mom, I always stopped by McDonald's for a berry smoothie. And though she always requested their latest *collectible* trinket, the smoothie was all she got. Lucky for me, her disappointment melted with her first slurp of that chilly delight. While her lips never left the flexible straw, her curious eyes followed me as I carried load after load of materials past her as she sat in her red reclining chair.

"What's going on?" she asked.

"I'm renovating your house."

She furrowed her brow. "Who's paying for all that?"

"You are. So, cheer up. You may have to go back to work," I said.

Every subsequent trip to Home Depot sparked the same conversation.

I kept her apprised of my progress and involved her in paint and carpet color decisions. We chose light coffee for the walls, white for the windows, doors, and trim. When it came time to choose the new carpet, I placed two three-by-three-inch samples on her lunch tray and left the room to refill her sippy cup. When I returned, she had a carpet sample in her mouth and a scowl on her face.

"This is not a cookie."

I stifled a laugh. "No, it's a carpet sample. Which one tastes better?"

She chose well.

Next up, the vestibule with a new design inside and out, new front door, new sidelights, new doorbell. To spice up the curb appeal, I painted the door bright green. My brothers gave me a lot of grief about that door, but I picked its unique color for three reasons. One: it was the only bright-green door in town. Two: it matched the foliage in the front garden. Three, and most importantly: Mom loved it.

After completing final touches, I first carried Mom down to the basement to see what all that fuss was about. I'm not sure how much of the old basement she remembered, but she loved the new one. We marked the event with a photo of her sitting on the new coffee-colored couch with a mini keg of Newcastle Brown Ale on her lap. I snapped another photo with her on a treadmill in the new man cave. She seemed happy to be back on her feet and exercising, but her extended middle finger squeezing the safety rail suggested otherwise.

I then carried her upstairs to christen the new bathroom with a bubble bath—her first in years. But a near tragedy cut the celebration short when she passed out in the tub.

Great. I try to do a nice thing and I kill my mother, I thought. At least she smelled good.

I dried her off, put her to bed, and called a nurse. She said leaving Mom in the hot bath for too long caused her blood pressure to drop, which caused her to faint. I kept watch over her until she woke up half an hour later. Mom didn't remember passing out, but she did remember the new bathroom, so it was a win-win for me. However, there would be no more bubble baths.

My two-year project was nearly complete. Only the first-floor bathroom remained, but due to unforeseen circumstances that would have to wait. Our home was once again a warm and welcoming place for everyone to enjoy, just like the one I grew up in.

If you rebuild it, they will return, and return they did. Friends and family visited more often. And once again we celebrated Thanksgiving, Christmas, Easter, and birthday dinners, which all took on new meaning.

CHAPTER 38

Day of Beauty

Mom wakes in a tizzy.

Mom: I have no idea what my hair looks
like to go out in public.

It needs to be set.

Me: When are you going out in public?

Mom: I don't know.

(She falls back asleep.)

In the past, my mother had always taken pride in her overall appearance, but as a former hand model, she took particular pride in her fingernails. She wore them long and natural. No gels or acrylics for her, and they were always painted red. To keep them looking good, she treated herself to weekly manicures at the beauty parlor. As a ten-year-old budding artist, she even let me try my hand at painting her precious nails once or twice, but most likely a day or two before a professional restored their beauty. Still, how a working mother of six kept them in such fine shape between manicures was nothing short of a miracle. And as far back as I can remember, the compliments flooded in.

Though she never sacrificed her long nails for motherhood, she did her long locks. Shampoos and sets became the new norm. Occasionally, she'd spice things up with a perm and frosting that required a reintroduction to her family. Even the dog needed a second sniff. But one was enough for me. I donned a clothespin to stomach that pungent, chemical cloud swirling about her head.

Hoping to preserve her investment, she wrapped her new 'do' in pink hair tape at bedtime. But more often than not, the tape instead stuck her head to the pillow. And although the battle to free herself often defeated the tape's intended purpose, this ritual continued for years. And like Dad, Mom was a recycler. I'd often find a curly strand or two of hair clinging to the surviving bands of pink tape stuck to her bedroom mirror, happy to live another day.

Beginning in the 1990s, whenever Mom visited me on the West Coast, I took her to my friend Stan's Beverly Hills salon for the movie-star treatment where she sat in the same chair that Betty White sat in for her movie-star treatment. They'd crossed paths only once, but Mom really liked Betty, and who didn't? She wanted an autograph, but my mother, who was sociable on any other day, hesitated. Lucille Ball had snapped at her fifty years earlier and forever lost a fan. So, Mom asked the receptionist for help. Betty, being "Betty," of course obliged, and my mother returned home with a cherished memento.

Highlights in Hollywood occurred so often during her trips, they came to be expected: witnessing me in action on the set of *Days of Our Lives*, meeting Gladys Knight and the Pips as they filmed their latest music video, eating lunch with Bob Hope sitting in the next booth. And let's not forget bumping into Erik Estrada, semi-hidden behind his Ray-Ban Aviators, in the dairy section at my local Ralph's Grocery where he greeted us with his patented "Hey."

The streak of our Hollywood highlights

nearly ended in 1992. But after several uneventful days, the Rodney King riots erupted and saved my derriere. Except she mistook the looting for bargain hunting and, as usual, my shopaholic mother wanted to partake.

Now Mom's trips to the beauty parlor were but a distant memory. So, I launched the Day of Beauty to recreate that weekly pampering she so loved, and I'm sure, so sorely missed. I initially scheduled it on Sundays, but when my once-a-Catholic-always-a-Catholic mother objected, I promptly moved it to Saturdays. Eternity in hell averted.

The Day of Beauty evolved into its own multitasking operation. While Mom did her business on the commode, and depending on how long she took, I performed many of the chores on the DOB menu: a full sponge bath, soaking her feet in Epsom salts, shampoo, condition, and rinse—Mom's least favorite part. Even though I warmed the water, covered her in towels, and worked fast, she shivered every time and accompanied those shivers with quivers of *oohs*. Was the risk of pneumonia worth it? I thought so. She smelled good and her hair looked great.

One day, hoping to make Mom's adventures on the commode a tad more pleasant, I offered her a cup of hot tea with skim milk, no sugar. It was a hit. And from that day forward, a cup of tea on the commode became a staple on the menu.

Once Mom finished her tea, we would move to the bed where I attended to any pressing medical needs followed by a massage with body lotion. After sprinkling baby powder, securing a new diaper, donning a fresh nightdress *of her choosing*, we got to my favorite part: our morning hug, which neither of us ever wanted to end. Then I would brush and blow-dry her hair as she sat in her wheelchair. Ponytails were the norm, but on special occasions I braided her hair, which had once again grown long. Lessons learned growing up with three sisters with equally long locks came in handy.

Next on the menu: her treasured fingernails. Removing old nail polish posed no problem. However, what followed did. During my childhood, I only questioned my mother's love on two occasions: when she served her tuna casserole, and when she pushed back my cuticles. She deemed it a necessary evil. As a kid, I did not. I found clever ways to avoid her casserole, but never the cuticle torture. The thought alone still makes me cringe. Now with the tool in the other hand, the temptation to inflict some degree of payback on my dear mother was almost too much to resist. But resist I did.

Instead, I saved my energy for my next challenge: trimming those prized possessions. I had to be tactful, knowing she'd fight even the slightest pruning. And fight she did. But being at the mercy of a persistent itch from chronic pruritus and showing no self-control, those long and dangerous nails had to go. When charm failed, I resorted to guilt-tripping.

"Mom, Momma, look at me please. Before you stands your strong and vibrant son who will be nothing but an empty shell of his former self, and whose soul will surely burn in hell if you scratched yourself with those things, drew blood, got an infection, became critically ill, or worse, and I didn't do everything in my power to prevent it. Is that what you want for me?"

Okay, a bit dramatic. Mom could shatter my heart with just a look. But hey, it worked. My oh-so-stubborn mom yielded. They say Jewish mothers invented guilt, but Catholic mothers perfected it. Well, I learned from one of Our Lady of Mount Carmel's guilt-tripping best. However, the epic battle to render her nails to a harmless length took several more Days of Beauty—rivaled only by the long, drawn-out surrender of her old, tattered tissues. Gracious in defeat, Mom offered her expertise.

"That's not how you do it. File in one direction."

I dutifully obeyed, then topped them off with a bright-red nail polish to match her soon-to-be bright-red lips.

Lucky for me, a podiatrist tackled Mom's toenails. No clippers on earth posed any threat to those thick, funky biological wonders. Only Dr. Arnold and his weapon of choice—an electric grinder—stood a chance. I can't say he won, but he did the best he could. So, let's call it a draw.

On the inaugural Day of Beauty, after completing all of my tasks, I parked Mom's wheelchair in front of the large dining room mirror, leaned in cheek to cheek, and asked, "Who's that pretty girl?"

She gazed in awe at her reflection. When

her eyes lit up and she smiled her approval, my heart melted. How long had it been since someone treated her special? How long had it been since she looked in a mirror and liked what she saw? How long had it been since she truly felt beautiful? Why do we think these basic human needs fade with time? Day of Beauty's profound power was a revelation. I made sure we stopped at that mirror every Saturday, and all the days in between. And every time I leaned in cheek to cheek and asked, "Who's that pretty girl?" my mother beamed.

CHAPTER 39

Genevieve's Personal Chef

Me: Caryl called. Says she's bringing soup.
Mom: I hope it's better than Michael's.

O ther than Michael's Potluck Tuesdays, the occasional sushi night, or the obligatory monthly takeout from Boston Market, I cooked all of Mom's meals. A task not without its perils. This woman whose taste buds retired years ago still had a particularly picky palate. I don't know whether it was the color or texture, but she could be brutal. Meals on Wheels failed to satisfy her, and so did two out of the three live-in caretakers. Even Michael's one-meal-a-week was a crapshoot. As soon as Mom spotted his Crock-Pot, she scolded him.

"Not your soup again!"

I got my first taste of the Simon Cowell of home cooking when I served a breakfast dish she hadn't eaten in years. Then I dared to ask, "Best French toast ever?"

She forced a smile and shook her head. For the record, I make excellent French toast.

Luckily for me, I was a pretty good cook before taking this job. I grew up watching both of my parents in the kitchen. I even took cooking lessons as a child. But don't take my word for it.

Years ago, while researching for a new packaging project in the cookware section of Macy's, a graphic design colleague and I naturally started discussing food. Upon hearing about my culinary specialties, he joked, "You'll make a good wife one day. Wanna get married?"

I laughed, but the lady eavesdropping in the next aisle turned white. Understandable, as it was Columbus, Ohio, in 1983.

Determined to win Mom over and avoid any more of her ego-crushing, I tried to keep things exciting. I made sure all meals were prepared and served with love. Oatmeal was her go-to breakfast, but she also liked eggs: omelets, scrambled, or poached, served with

homemade hash browns. My French toast—
secret ingredient: a dash of vanilla extract—
became a Sunday morning favorite, whether she
admitted it or not. For a healthy touch, I always
included a side of fresh fruit. For lunch, I served
a variety of sandwiches or soups with fruit,
salad, or coleslaw. If she wasn't terribly hungry,
just a snack would do. Dinner was the most
challenging and time-consuming. Whipping
up my world-famous ratatouille, emphasizing
the "world-famous" part, catapulted this
healthy meal onto Mom's list of favorites. My
homemade chicken soup and many of my pasta
dishes also made the list. She loved spareribs, so
I bought a grill to barbeque them all year round.
Mom loved fresh corn on the cob, but getting
the corn off the cob was difficult with her loose
dentures that she refused to let me secure. So I
stripped those kernels off with a knife like my
babysitter did for me many years ago. Thank
you, Mrs. Becker.

Mom's lasagna was my all-time favorite dish.
Growing up, I often offered to help, or at least
pretended to. The aroma of succulent ground
sirloin, fresh garlic, seasoned salt, and black
pepper seduced my taste buds every time. While

she focused on making her savory tomato sauce, I couldn't resist swiping spoonfuls of meat from the easily poachable pan. Chalking up the losses to "quality control" did not pass muster with my "I'm from Missour-uh" Mom, since my *control* was spotty at best. After promising to behave, she let me stay. I watched and learned from the master.

While the noodles boiled, she combined the meat, the sauce, and a secret blend of herbs and spices. She then layered the noodles, sauce, ricotta, and mozzarella cheese in a deep pan and topped it with a blanket of freshly grated parmesan. I would peek through the tiny oven window as it baked and bubbled, and not yanking that door open and digging in was another test of self-control. But the greater test would come twenty minutes later as it cooled, unguarded on the stovetop. Where this Irish girl learned how to make this classic Italian dish remains a mystery. But those who had been lucky enough to taste it experienced heaven on earth.

Over the years, I had experimented with vegetarian versions, but I wanted to recreate the magic of the original for Mom. I also resumed my poaching, so I cooked plenty of extra meat to cover my losses. The first time I served it, she looked it over for a moment or two before plunging her fork into the near-crispy parmesan crust that released a familiar whiff of bliss. As she chewed, her long-absent taste buds came alive, confirmed by her ear-to-ear grin. My—or rather, her own—lasagna also made the list.

Though tempted when she misbehaved, I never cooked Mom's all-time worst meal: her way-too-salty, blood-pressure-raising tuna casserole topped with crushed potato chips. I questioned her love for us every time she served it. I didn't want her to question mine, so I never served tuna casserole.

My respect for all moms and dads who provide and prepare a full daily menu for their children year after year grew tenfold during my short time at it, but it wasn't always a rosy picture. Mom's iron will reared its ugly head from time to time. I did my best, but charm, guilt, and my lack of parenting prowess had its limits. Mom usually devoured everything I prepared, but that night, without explanation, she refused. I pleaded.

"You need to eat to keep up your strength."

No response.

"Can you please tell me why?"

Still no response.

"I turned my life upside down to come here and take care of you. I do everything: cook, clean, wipe your butt. You need to show some appreciation and eat your dinner."

She didn't budge.

I threw my hands up, flicked off the lights, and marched down to the basement, leaving her alone in the dark.

After taking out my frustrations on an innocent load of laundry—jamming it in the washer, drenching it with liquid detergent, and slamming the lid down on it—I calmed down a bit and returned to the kitchen for round two.

When I switched the lights back on, my heart sank. Mom was sitting in silence with her hands folded in her lap. Her knife and fork rested on an empty plate. She'd eaten her entire dinner in the dark. Not easy at any age. And once again, she'd out-guilt-tripped me.

When we had previous run-ins, she had no problem expressing her disapproval with a sharp look or a comment like, "I don't like you swearing." But her silent treatment made my this-is-going-to-hurt-me-more-than-it-hurts-you parental cliché actually come true.

Lost for words, I just leaned in, kissed her on the cheek, and whispered, "Thank you."

CHAPTER 40

Un Maniaque du Ménage

Mom: Oh, you are here.

*Me: Of course I'm here. Where else
am I going to be?*

Mom: Just wanted to make sure.

Me: That's all you wanted?

As a teenager, whenever I visited my grandmother, a foul combination of sweat, urine, gas, and bad breath greeted and gagged me as soon as I entered her house. I didn't know any better. I thought it was just part of getting old. That "senior smell" seemed to linger in all old people's homes.

Well, I didn't want that in Mom's.

To keep her fresh and clean and smelling like a daisy, I gave her full sponge baths in the morning and at night. I changed and washed her clothes and bedding often, and in addition to keeping the entire house clean, I installed commercial air fresheners.

Okay, I admit I'm a clean freak, a bit anal-retentive, or as they call me in France, *un maniaque du ménage*. Everyone who set foot in my home understood. Many poked fun at me, but of all the flaws to be teased about, being "too neat" ain't too bad.

When friends in Los Angeles first met my parents, they often asked, "Who did he get that neat thing from?"

Mom and Dad shrugged off any responsibility, yet they and my five siblings—whether deli-berate or not—all contributed to me being a clean freak. Growing up in a family of eight with both parents working full time, the house got messy, and things got lost, especially when my siblings and I didn't do our chores. My stubborn streak—Mom and Dad couldn't shrug that off—reared its ugly head when I finally had enough and refused to tackle the mountain of dishes after dinner. "You will never find a sink full of dirty dishes in my house," I said to my father. I've never broken that promise. In fact, when I'm alone, I clean most of my pots, pans, and dishes before I sit down to eat. This might seem a bit too much, but there's a practical reason. I can enjoy my meal and not worry about a disaster to contend with afterward.

The never-ending cleaning war eased up when *you know who* moved out, but one last battle remained. On Michael's Potluck Tuesdays, he often left a mess in his wake. To be fair, he attempted to clean the pots, the dishes, the counters, the table, the floor, and the stove. But as I can be a bit anal about these things, it took me longer to clean up after his attempt than if he'd made no attempt at all. So, to avoid future Tuesday night fights, we—me more than he—decided that Michael cooked, and I cleaned.

CHAPTER 41

And as Swift as Evolution, She Shuffled Across the Floor

Mom: Why am I always in bed?
Why don't you let me out?

Me: Mom, you can't walk.

Mom: Maybe I could if you put down the railing.

Me: You haven't walked in a year.

Mom's best friend, Mary, once told me, "Your mother is the bravest woman I've ever known." When Mom was in her midtwenties and sick and tired of cavities, she demanded her dentist remove all of her teeth in a single session, and without any novocaine. Against his better judgment, he yielded. Mary had held Genevieve's hand through the entire "procedure" . . . if you can call it that. That trip to the dentist sounded more like a torture scene from a horror film without the benefit of surprise for the victim. I thought I had a high-pain threshold, but that was off the charts.

"She never complained," Mary said.

I can't even imagine.

Now this brave woman seemed perfectly content to waste away in her sedentary lifestyle, but I was not. With a little encouragement, she agreed to get moving again. We played card games, bingo, and even Angry Birds on her iPad. We did daily arm exercises. She helped with the laundry. While I folded sheets and shirts, she folded the socks and towels with precision and care. During morning and evening shifts, she washed her face, underarms, and privates, in that order, with me rinsing the washcloth in between.

We did have some bumps early on. I caught her trying to wash her face *after* scrubbing her privates. One time, she wouldn't pucker up for ChapStick, which was unusual since this kissing bandit puckered up for everything else.

"Maybe you'll have better luck," I said as I handed it to her. When she coated everything but her lips, I snatched it back. "Okay, maybe not."

Another time she nearly used her roll-on deodorant on her already dry lips. I quickly learned, like with a baby, you can't turn away, not even for a second.

These activities all led up to our biggest challenge: walking again. Her legs were still strong. She proved that during every trip to the commode, but it had been more than a year since she'd walked. To my surprise, she jumped at the chance. Well, she would have if she could have.

Mom, clad in her new non-slip socks, sat on the edge of the bed.

"Are you ready?" I asked.

She nodded a cautious yes.

I started the countdown. "One, two, three, up." I held her tightly as she rose. "Don't worry, I got you. Take it nice and easy."

Supporting her own full weight, she dragged one foot in front of the other on her way to the wheelchair a few feet away. Before that day, even that distance seemed impossible. Aside from being bedridden all those months, she had a bad hip—two, in fact—and the replaced hip gave her the most trouble. But determined not to let either of us down, she muscled through. She slowly shuffled across the floor. When we reached the finish line, she turned and landed in the chair with a thud and let out a heavy sigh. We celebrated with a high-five.

As Mom gained strength, her shuffles became steps. Within a month, she walked—with my help—from her bed all the way to the kitchen. She worked her way up to five days a week, sometimes six, but being a good Catholic girl, she always rested on the seventh.

CHAPTER 42

Does Wiping Butt Cause Amnesia?

Now, what is it I call you? —Mom

To boost Mom's spirits and keep her socially active, Michael signed her up for Senior Connections back in 2009. Though it sounded more like a dating site, the only dating happening there was of the expiration kind. Most members played cards or competitive bingo all—day—long. Some sat in front of the television as *Wheel of Fortune* droned on at an ear-piercing volume. Others just drooled while dozing off in a corner. The slogan, "Misery loves company," would all but guarantee a steady stream of customers, forever. Mom put up with it five days a week by gravitating toward the rare members who were still with it. For her, it served as a welcome diversion from the Tweedles.

On a surprise visit home, I stopped by to check the place out. It was a good day. Mom was in a good mood, and they were celebrating a member's eighty-sixth birthday. The birthday girl bragged nonstop in her several-packs-a-day raspy voice about her sons and only her sons.

"My boys, my boys, I just love my boys. They're the best."

She all but ignored her crestfallen daughter standing at her side. I later learned that not only did that forgotten girl care for her mother 24/7, but she also created Senior Connections specifically for her.

Now I wondered was this my fate, to step up and take care of my mother's every need only to be ignored or, worse, forgotten? That could never happen, not to me, not by *my* mom. I was the one who cooked, fed, and dressed her. I changed diapers, bathed, and baby powdered her. I combed her hair, trimmed her fingernails, brushed her teeth—in Mom's case, dentures. I carried, chauffeured, and shopped. I cleaned, washed, and folded laundry. I ordered and administered vitamins and medications. I comforted and cajoled and hugged and kissed. I cheered her up doing the Riverdance Irish jig, which made her laugh but my shins cry. I got her out of bed and walking again. I navigated road trips and invented Day of Beauty. I celebrated her every success on the commode. And I was the one who performed, with tender loving care, my least favorite task, and perhaps Mom's as well: wiping her butt.

In King Henry VIII's day, the Groom of the Stool was a coveted position. The physical intimacy gained him much confidence with the king, which led to the sharing of many royal secrets, which afforded the groom a certain amount of sway with his master. And though there were, undoubtedly, some downsides to the job, the Groom of the Stool never feared the king would ever forget his name. So, surely, my mother would never forget mine. But one morning, after serving her breakfast in bed, she greeted me with:

Mom: Now, what is it I call you?

At first, I thought she was joking—she had a wicked sense of humor—but the look on her face confirmed she was not.

Me: Really? You don't remember me?

She shook her head.

Me: Name your children.

Mom: *(rattling them off)* Laurel, Michael, Caryl, David, Deecy.

Me: And?

Stumped, she shrugged.

Me: *(crestfallen)* Mark.

Mom: Oh. Mark with a k?

Me: Yes, Mark with a k. Your favorite son.

Mom: I don't have favorites.

Me: *(under my breath)* You have a favorite to forget.

How dare she. My own mother. And she showed absolutely no remorse. To help relieve her of her clear *lack* of guilt, I printed my name, "M-A-R-K," in large Helvetica Bold letters, and taped it to the ceiling. I left off the "Your favorite son" part, a decision I would soon regret.

It proved to be a useful memory tool. Whenever I entered her room, she'd say, "Hi . . ." and after a glance up at my visual aid, she proudly finished with, "Mark."

All good.

Other days, when she forgot to look up, I'd get only a blank stare. It evolved into a game.

If she snuck a peek, I'd call her on it. "You cheated."

"I did not," she'd protest.

"Then what's my name?"

Mom wrestled with her memory until she could no longer resist. Her eyes shot skyward, and with a sly yet relieved smile, she answered, "Mark." When I threatened to take down the paper with my name to avoid further temptation, she mulled it over before saying, "Don't."

Problem solved, but not the underlying one. Out of Mom's six kids, I was the only one she forgot. I was also the only one who regularly wiped her butt. So, by deductive reasoning, and I hope science one day proves me right that wiping butts causes amnesia. Now let me be clear, I'm not talking about wiping your own butt. Imagine the chaos if wiping your own butt caused memory loss. People might never find their way out of the bathroom. I'm talking about a caregiver-patient relationship involving wiping the butt of another.

So, if you believe my theory to be credible, and you currently wipe a loved one's butt or plan to in the future and want to avoid my misery, post your name in large block letters in a conspicuous place, or wear a name tag.

CHAPTER 43

Just the Two of Us

Bring warm clothing.
It's bitter cold out here. —Mom

'Twas the night before Christmas . . . no, 'twas the night of Christmas. The first without Dad, or the second. Things got hazy after his passing. I'd flown in from the Left Coast to spend the holidays in New Jersey where it was bitter cold outside and warm and toasty inside, just as it should be during this time of year. It's quite often the opposite in Los Angeles, which made it tough to get into the spirit of things.

Mom's house was decorated as usual: the tree, the Nativity scene, the stockings. Even with one less stocking on this Noël, they still crowded the fireplace. But there were none of her mouthwatering cookies. No homemade apple, cherry, or pumpkin pies. I guess it was too soon to embrace the new normal.

We celebrated Christmas Eve at David's house: his family, Michael's family, Mom, and me. We all did our best to keep the mood merry. I hoped the tumblers of holiday cheer would help, but they didn't.

On Christmas Day, David and Michael were off celebrating with their families. My three sisters, who lived far away, celebrated with theirs. This left Mom and me on our own. We filled the hours as best we could. We attended Mass at Our Lady of Mount Carmel. Lit a candle for Dad. Exchanged gifts. Fielded phone calls. But with an empty house and the mood understandably less festive, we decided to brave the elements and go out to a fancy restaurant for our Christmas dinner.

However, spontaneity had its drawbacks. Many of our local favorites were closed, others fully booked. We felt like Mary and Joseph desperately looking for a room at the inn. As the sun fell from the sky, we ventured outside of our village. Still no luck. The holiday spirit quickly lost its charm.

Then, in perhaps a flash of divine intervention, the neon lights of the Suburban Diner, an eatery where my sister waited tables long ago, appeared. Surely, they would have room for us as well as all the other poor souls who found themselves alone on Christmas night. They did, and they welcomed us with open arms.

Our server—a lifer, I imagine—led us to one of several empty booths. Other than "What will it be?" she asked no questions, though I'm sure she had a few. Once we settled in, I scanned the room, hoping not to see a familiar face. How could I explain that our loved ones forgot about us on this of all nights? But we Porros did not like to impose or bother anyone, not even family. Mom and I sat alone, and we made the most of it, just like we Porros always did. We enjoyed each other's company, we ate a fine Suburban Diner dinner, and we topped it off with a slice of homemade pumpkin pie—not as good as Mom's, but good enough. And though this might not have been the ideal scenario for our Christmas night, I wouldn't have missed it for the world.

CHAPTER 44

Queen for a Day

Mom: Why do you treat me so well?

Me: Because you deserve to be treated like a queen.
(She burps.)

But queens don't do that.

Mom: How do you know?

One morning, a strange ringing sound woke me from my well-earned and much-needed sleep. I hopped out of bed, bounded down the stairs, and marched into my mother's room where I found her sitting up in bed, striking the perfect Queen Elizabeth pose. A tiny brass bell dangled between her regal fingertips. I stared at her in disbelief.

Me: Please tell me you didn't ring that to summon me.

Mom: I most certainly did.

Me: And now I will take that lovely little bell from you and officially retire it, so it never rings again.

Mom: For heaven's sake, why?

Me: Because you are not the queen, and I am not your servant. You are my mother. I am your son, who is here out of love, not duty.

She reluctantly handed me the bell.

Me: So, Your Majesty, what do you desire on this bright, musical morning?

Mom: I'd like some tea.

Me: *(coaching her)* Please.

Mom: *(she teases a royal smile)* Please.

Me: Would you like that now, or shall we wait until you ascend the throne? *(gesturing to the commode.)*

Mom: Now, please.

Me: As you wish.

Mom enjoyed playing the queen, if only for that one day. She'd always loved being pampered at the beauty parlor, and now by me. She bathed in it, but at times, she overdid the royalty bit. God forbid she found her Bichon Frisé blanket or grandson Josh's photo a tiny bit out of place. Her regal lips remained silent while her imperial finger did the talking. Commanding up an eighth of an inch here, down a quarter of an inch there, and so on, until perfection ruled. This exercise in patience got old fast. It was enough to pray for blindness.

In contrast, Dad had always felt guilty about bothering anyone, and did so only when absolutely necessary, and he often apologized after. During his final days, he never cried out for help or rang an annoying brass bell. Instead, he put what he needed to song and hoped for the best. His delightful ditty went something like this:

"I'm just lying here in my bed waiting for somebody to help me get to the toilet since I can't get up on my own. So, I'll keep singing this song until someone comes along so I can do my business in the proper place . . ."

The first time I heard him singing, I selfishly listened for way too long before coming to his aid. It was so damn entertaining I didn't want it to end.

Though Mom lacked royal blood, she did possess many royal qualities. She kept her emotions from the public eye, remained stoic when facing adversity, and never complained of pain. She didn't swear—a fact we all took pride in, and one trait I had yet to master.

One frustrating day, I let loose with a few *choice* words. Knowing how much cursing upset her, I said, "Sorry, Mom. It's hard being a parent."

"I guess, but *I* never swore," she replied.

So true, even when she had good reason to. One time, when Mom was shuttling my high school friends home, a car had cut her off.

"Fudgie wudgie," she muttered.

My friends snickered in the back seat, thinking she kept it clean for them.

"That wasn't for your benefit," I explained. "That's as bad as it gets."

Neither of my parents swore. When Mom got mad, she'd say, "Nincompoop, I'm fed up," or if absolutely furious, "I'm so angry I could spit." When Dad got angry, it seemed like food came to mind. He said things like "Chowderhead," "You're full of soup," or he replaced "hell" with his favorite meat: "Get the ham out of here."

In the company of the Christians in my family, I worked hard to curtail my cursing. One night, while dashing through the snow to catch Christmas service, my young, impressionable nephews and I lagged way behind their mother, a former track star. Frustrated by how fast she was and how fast we weren't, I started to say my favorite swear word. "Mutha . . ." but for my nephews' benefit, I finished with, "Followers. We're mutha-followers." Saved! I got away with it because that was what we were at that moment.

My Queen Mother's other royal qualities included being faithful to her husband and equally devoted to her children, whether or not she remembered their names. She once hired a maid to keep her palace clean, but that maid had done little of that and disappeared after a few weeks. I believe she ran off with some of the crown jewels, yet Mom refused to speak ill of her. Our queen also took to her grave, no matter how many times I'd asked, "Which cousin stole your father's prized gun collection?"

Even though I retired the queen's tiny brass bell that day, my mother still reigned over this castle. And I, her humble servant—on most occasions—sucked it up and did what I could to fulfill all of Her Majesty's wishes. I also prayed that all my future foul language fell on deaf ears.

CHAPTER 45

Genevieve and the "Two Gs"

Mom calls out in the middle of the night.
I fly down the stairs and slide into her room.

Mom: I need to lose some weight.

Me: Why?

Mom: I'm not eating right.

Me: You're eating fine. If anything,
you're not eating enough.

Mom: Well, whatever it is, I need to do
something about it.

(She falls back to sleep.)

Whether it was Mom and her endless snacks or Dad dusting off his well-worn corny jokes, childhood friends loved coming over to our house because my parents were so much fun. They each possessed their own unique sense of humor. Dad was the puncher. Mom was more of a counterpuncher. But the stress and strain of a long and difficult marriage took its toll and stifled much of my parents' true personalities in their later years. However, when they were out of the house and away from one another, they shined. Each was charming, engaging, and funny.

Whenever Dad visited me, he always said, "I'm easy to get along with."

And he was. Mom was too.

Fortunately, the genetic gods passed down some of their wit and humor to me, and it, among other pluses, proved to be a lifesaver. When promoting Grandpa Po's Originals at a Whole Foods Market in West Hollywood, a young man attempted to down the entire sample cup of the crunchy golden nuggets in one gulp and started choking.

I leaned in and whispered, "You're gonna kill my business if you die here. Can you do it over in produce?"

He burst out laughing and spit out a hull. I saved his life, and he bought two bags in gratitude.

One of my favorite lines from Dad came after his many attempts at being a good and caring uncle to the daughter of his deceased brother. When she earned her bachelor's and master's degrees, he sent cards and checks but received no response. When she got married, he wasn't invited but sent a card and check, and again received no response. To celebrate the birth of her only daughter, he sent yet another card and check. And once again, received no response, prompting him to declare, "That was the last time I never heard from her."

Mom didn't try to be funny; she just was.

An absolute classic "Genevieve" comedy moment came during a business trip to Silicon Valley in the early 1990s. Mom was visiting me in Los Angeles, so I took her up north. After the meeting, we ate lunch at a local diner with my friends, Cindy and Cathy. Somehow the conversation drifted to G-string bathing suits (or as I call them, "anal floss"). We talked about their popularity and who would—or who should not—be jumping on that fashion bandwagon.

Mom was completely in the dark. "What's a G-string?" she asked.

The girls described them in detail.

"G-string," Mom replied. "I'd need two Gs."

Cindy and Cathy spilled out of the booth and onto the floor, roaring with laughter. And my mom forever cemented her status as a comedy hero.

CHAPTER 46

Superstorm Sandy

*Hurricane Sandy was among the most costly
natural disasters in US history,
causing more than $70 billion in damage.*
—*Encyclopedia Britannica*

To get a jump start on every project, my boss at the Corporate Design Center taught me to panic early. In reality, this just fed on itself and created an endless panic loop, which meant working all-nighters until the job was done. I only escaped, and got a good night's sleep, by leaving the company. But I still believed the concept had merit. Years later, that sleep-deprived experience paid big dividends when dealing with Superstorm Sandy.

As October 29, 2012 approached, I panicked early and ordered an Eton portable storm radio. It came equipped with an emergency light and a hand crank to recharge my iPhone. When my arm nearly fell off testing its charging capability, I prayed for no power outages for my arm's sake.

To play it safe, I dashed off to Home Depot and discovered I wasn't the only one who believed my old boss's concept had merit. The run-on flashlights and batteries in all shapes and sizes left me with slim pickings. I bought a multipack of mini lights and enough batteries to power their mighty but eerie glow—more suitable for a night of scary storytelling than calming my fragile ninety-year-old mother. But I had her care routine down to a tee, and if forced, I could do it in the dark.

Even though we were far enough inland to not worry about flooding from the surging Atlantic, I had plenty of other concerns: high winds, flying debris, and downed power lines, all magnified due to Mom's age and immobility. To keep her safe, I set up a temporary bedroom in the newly renovated basement. I placed her old reclining bed in the corner, away from all windows.

On the day of the storm, I brought down the commode and all the necessary items to sustain us for a few days. I parked my Prius between houses to protect it from the wind, falling branches, or—God forbid—an uprooted tree. Then I carried Mom down to her new digs. At first she was content, but as time clicked away, discomfort gained ground, shedding no doubt on just how critical her pulsating air mattress was. Stuffing extra pillows under Mom's knees, rolling her on her side, and adjusting the bed up and down provided only temporary relief, but as usual, she toughed it out.

The winds picked up just after dark. The brunt of the storm hit around 8:00 p.m. Not too much rain, but howling winds soon blew down power lines, leaving us in the eerie glow of those mini lights. Then I heard a strange *whoosh* at the side of the house. Perhaps something outside fell, but it fell softly as if cushioned. I ran up the stairs to check. When I pointed a mini light through the kitchen window, I saw only leaves and branches. Peeking out the side door revealed even more leaves and branches, but they were attached to our now uprooted sixty-foot-tall Linden tree. It was the same tree I'd gotten stuck in as a kid and was rescued from by my dad, much to the amusement of the entire neighborhood. So I had mixed feelings about that tree. I wasn't sad that it fell, but rather *where* it fell: on top of my strategically placed Prius. I had to wait for daylight to assess the full extent of the damage or make any plans for a proper automotive funeral.

Morning brought welcome relief. The winds died down, and our electricity powered back up. As soon as it was safe, I returned Mom to her bedroom and to the comfort of her "sorely" missed pulsating air mattress. Then I grabbed a saw, took a deep breath, and went in search of my Prius, buried deep within the jungle that now occupied our driveway.

I hacked through the tangled green mass and was surprised and relieved to find my car relatively unscathed. The low slope of our garage roof broke the tree's fall, suspending the trunk and the bulk of its weight. My Prius was resting comfortably below the Linden canopy with only a few scratches. Strategically placed indeed.

Unlike many others on the East Coast, our family lucked out. Mom and I weathered the storm with a sore back, a fallen tree, and a few scratches on my car. David, just a mile away, lost power for over a week. A kind neighbor with a generator and a long extension cord helped soften the blow. Caryl, who lived at the Jersey Shore, fared even better: no flooding, no power outage, no fallen trees. Sandy hit Michael the hardest—not the storm, but the wrath inflicted by our persnickety neighbor. He blamed Michael—not Mother Nature—for our fallen tree, much of which landed in his yard. But Mother Nature didn't have a chain saw. So, to calm "Hurricane Ed" before *he* transformed into a superstorm, Michael took out his wrath on that Linden tree.

CHAPTER 47

Why Are You Doing This?

Honor thy father and thy mother. —God

I never believed in angels, but for some reason they believed in me, and I'm truly thankful for it. They kept watch over me during the many crazy, death-defying stunts I indulged in as a kid. I hopped on freight and passenger trains, and—only after learning the hard way—made sure to hit the ground running when hopping off. Still, chances were, momentum slammed me ass-first onto the sidewalk. Not cracking my skull was a good day. I crawled through dark, dank sewer pipes, never knowing where or if they ended, or what might be flowing or creeping my way. Thinking about tight spaces all these years later makes me cringe. For reasons I will never understand, my friends and I—fully clothed and in sneakers—would jump into the roaring rapids of the Hohokus River after a hard rain. We floated over waterfalls and around boulders while dodging logs and debris for what seemed like miles. The only escape before reaching the Atlantic Ocean was to grab hold of pricker bushes spilling over the riverbanks and pull our soggy, beaten, and now bloody selves to safety. We called it body surfing. Sane people, no doubt, called it something else. If my mom or dad caught wind of any of these escapades, they surely would have done what trains, sewers, or that raging river never could: put me out of their misery.

How my parents survived their "sixpack" of kids confounds me to this day. Seeing what they went through while only knowing a fraction of what we did played a big part in me not wanting, or having, children.

I came close once. It happened in the fall of 1984, soon after I moved to Los Angeles. We met at a Hollywood party. For fun, I assumed a French accent and poured glass after glass of French wine for her, others, and many for myself. I remember little of what happened after, but in the morning, she said my accent did the trick. I blamed the wine.

A few weeks later, I got a call with the news. She ended it with, "Daddy arranged everything, so not to worry."

I had no say in the matter. I guess I could have, but staying quiet seemed right at the time.

And there I was some thirty years later embracing "parenthood." Only this time the child was my ninety-year-old mother. I jumped in with gusto and happily took on all of the usual first-time parent duties. I lost sleep . . . lots and lots of sleep.

The physical tasks, though time-consuming, were manageable, and with practice became routine. They were nothing compared to the emotional roller coaster I found myself on. I didn't expect it. Didn't want it. Tried to ignore it. But it crept up on me as I realized this "child" would sleep more hours, not fewer. Her vocabulary would not increase but diminish to barely a word. She would never again walk on her own. Never outgrow her dependency. She would only continue to decline. And—most difficult—I had to accept the fact that I would not have her for much longer.

My mother's life was in my hands. I needed her to understand that.

"Do you trust me?" I asked.

"Yes," she whispered.

"Do you understand I will do everything in my power to keep you healthy and safe?"

She smiled and nodded.

"That means I'm in charge. And that means you must listen and obey me."

Her mood shifted in an instant. She looked me dead in the eye and puckered up her lips. I wasn't sure if this was a sign of surrender or one wishing me luck. I kissed her and hoped for the best.

After a particularly stressful day for the both of us, Mom shot me a curious look and asked, "Why are you doing this?"

I paused and took a deep breath. "Because it's an honor for a son to take care of his mother," I answered in all sincerity.

Taken aback, she replied, "It is?"

Her surprise stung me on many levels. I felt the need to reassure her. "Of course. How long did you take care of me?" I said. She was unconvinced, so I continued. "Who forgave me when I shelled all those lobster tails and turned your lovely New Year's presentation into a pile of white meat? And who forgave me when her expensive but noisy spoked hubcaps flew off her car after I tried to silence them with Vaseline? And who didn't tell Dad I was suspended for two days in the seventh grade for slamming the vice principal's door?"

And with that, she smiled.

But her question got me thinking. Why did I take this on? Why did I give up my carefree bachelor's life to move back in to my childhood home? Yes, I was in a position to help. I had no children, no pets, and no current relationship tying me to Los Angeles—at least none that I knew of. My acting career had stalled long ago. And after devoting fifteen years of blood, sweat, and plenty of tears to my organic popcorn business, Grandpa Po's Originals barely had a kernel of life left in it.

Perhaps the pain of overhearing my brother Michael channeling Dad's tirades about money played a role. Mom's careless spending continued to be an issue as long as telemarketers had access to her, and she had access to a credit card.

Maybe I did it for selfish reasons. I wanted more than the eight days I got with my dad.

Maybe I needed a win. I needed to accomplish something meaningful, which, at that point in my life, I felt that I hadn't. I was good at many things, but I never stuck with one long enough to excel above all others. I got bored and moved on. That was my MO. When I met my niece's new father-in-law at her wedding in Bermuda, he asked what I did for work.

"I started five nonprofit businesses," I said.

He looked at me like I was Jesus.

"None were intended to be," I added quickly.

We shared a good laugh and returned to our Dark 'n' Stormys.

Taking this on, perhaps the biggest challenge of my life, could be my saving grace. After all, it was my mom. She never once gave up on me. So, I committed myself not only to her but to my five siblings. They all put their trust in me, and no matter how difficult—physically, mentally, or emotionally—this journey became, I was determined not to let any of them down. This time there would be no moving on until she decided to move on.

But during those difficult times, I often asked myself the same question: "Why are you doing this?"

Then I'd see her smile, or I'd catch one of her witty comebacks, or I'd melt when she puckered up for a kiss, and I had my answer.

So, maybe those angels who'd saved me all those times had a plan all along. Do I believe in them now? I think I do.

CHAPTER 48

Bed, Bath, and Beyond

Me: You had your own big bowl of ice cream.

Why are you stealing mine?

Mom: You had plenty.

Me: So, you're helping me out?

Mom: Yes.

Me: You're too good to me.

Dry skin: something we can all look forward to in our Golden Years. As we age, our oil glands dry up, our skin becomes thinner, and it retains less moisture. The result? Itchy skin. Most seniors suffer from it. Though not a serious condition on its own, the itch-scratch cycle can lead to more irritation and, in some cases, infection.

Mom's battle with dry skin was severe and difficult to watch. To ease her pain, I experimented with several remedies to help control that seemingly impossible itch. I tried Benadryl pills and cream. I tested mild soaps and body lotions. I sampled hypoallergenic laundry detergents and fabric softeners. I installed a humidifier to keep both the air and her skin moist. I kept her hydrated with a bottomless sippy cup. But nothing seemed to work.

While the search for a solution continued, good old-fashioned scratching provided the temporary relief she desperately needed. Even after trimming her lethal-length nails and making her wear gloves, Mom could still do some serious damage. So, for her protection, I provided the relief. After her sponge bath, before the body lotion and baby powder, Mom told me where it itched, and I scratched the spot using a wet washcloth as a buffer. On one particularly itchy evening, my mother went beyond bed, beyond bath, and . . . just . . . beyond.

It's possible the red wine led her—a lifelong teetotaler—down that path. I always enjoyed a glass or two of Cabernet Sauvignon with dinner. When I began cooking for Mom, I offered her a glass. She liked it. Since she was only taking Digoxin at the time I thought, *what's the harm?* So, I added wine to her dinner menu.

However, shortly after, I noticed changes. Changes in her personality. Dark changes. She began cheating at cards, paying no attention to me sitting across the table witnessing every shady move. Then, after polishing off her bowl of coffee ice cream, she dipped into mine as soon as I turned my back. When caught red-handed, she replied, "You had plenty." But cheating and stealing—venial sins in the eyes of the Church—were nothing compared to how low she would go on that unforgettable night.

It began innocently enough. As usual, I wet a washcloth in warm water and began at her shoulders.

Mom: A little to the left.

Me: Here?

Mom: Yes. A little harder.

Me: Good?

Mom: Yeah. Lower.

Me: Okay.

Mom: Lower.

Me: Here?

Mom: Lower.

Me: Okay.

She continued directing me as I worked my way down her body. But when I reached her nether regions, all guidance stopped. So, I stayed and scratched and scratched. She moaned softly, then not so softly. Then her jaw dropped. Her face twisted. Her soft moans turned into groans, and her facial contortions turned impure.

I recoiled in horror. *Oh my God, oh my God. Am I pleasuring my mother? My ninety-one-year-old mother? My ninety-one-year-old Catholic mother?*

All signs screamed yes. *Holy shit!* This is not something a son should see, let alone *do*. And for Christ's sake, not to his own mother, his ninety-one-year-old mother, his ninety-one-year-old Catholic mother. The Catholic guilt was heavy enough, but I also had no interest in proving Freud right, or like Oedipus, sticking needles in my eyes.

Me: Mom, I can't do this.

I handed her the washcloth and stepped back. She immediately picked up where I left off, then slammed it into high gear. Each sinful stroke brought her closer and closer to total and unadulterated ecstasy. I turned away to protect my eyes, then uttered what may be a first for a son to say to his mother, his ninety-one-year-old mother, his ninety-one-year-old Catholic mother.

Me: Momma, stop. You're gonna go blind.

CHAPTER 49

My Conversation with God

*What it's like to be a parent: It's among
the hardest things you'll ever do, but in exchange,
it teaches you the meaning of unconditional love.*

—Nicholas Sparks, The Wedding[1]

I have to admit there were times—I can't say how many, but more than a few—during our journey where I did almost lose all hope. My "I-love-my-job" mantra didn't help, nor did substantial amounts of red wine. So, one night I decided to vent directly to the Man upstairs.

When You whispered to Mom, "Be patient," back in 2011, who were You really talking to? And more to the point, how patient did You mean?

---

[1] Nicholas Sparks, *The Wedding*, (New York: Grand Central Publishing, 2003).

Don't get me wrong, I'm glad Mom came back from the dead in a somewhat miraculous fashion, a phoenix rising from the ashes and all that. I had no qualms about giving up my carefree bachelor life to become a sleep-deprived, stressed-out parent at fifty-five. I did not rue the day I moved back to my childhood home to tolerate Tammy and the Tweedles for months, which shaved off several years of my life, or when I gave up sex for the most part, which I'm sure shaved off several more. I did not rue the day I sacrificed all of this to take care of the cooking, the cleaning, the cajoling, the wiping butt, the smells, and so much more for a mother who couldn't remember my name without a visual aid stuck to the bedroom ceiling. I regretted none of that. Not one bit. I did it freely and willingly.

But when You spoke to her that day, You didn't say anything to me, did You? No, You did not.

There are times—and forgive me for thinking this—that maybe this whole "I'm-dying" thing was a ploy. A ruse to get her kids to come back and rescue her, and I was the sucker who fell for it hook, line, and sinker.

"Be patient."

Okay fine, but how patient? Can I at least have a clue as to how long Mom is going to be here? I don't want to rush her or anything. I'd just like an idea. I do have a life, or I *did*. Not that she doesn't. She has a good life now, and I'm happy to have played a part in that.

Is this about my commitment issues? Like I'm the only one wary of second dates. I know I get bored easily and move on, but that's not the case here. I'm not bored with Mom, far from it. Rarely is there a dull moment. I'm just . . .

Unconditional love, is that what this is all about? To teach me this "concept"? Let me tell you, I know all about unconditional love. I might not have a wife or children, or a girlfriend, but I had pets. Pets I loved unconditionally, as long as they obeyed. Same thing, right?

And I unconditionally accept the fact that I was partially responsible for the untimely death of my hamster when his tiny box roller-coastered off the side of my guitar case. Okay, maybe fully responsible. It broke my heart when Dad put him in that jar with that ether-soaked shred of terrycloth. I so wanted to crack the lid open and wake him, but I knew it would only prolong his suffering. How's that for some unconditional love?

And my dog Gina—well, she was Caryl's until she got bored, then mine until I got bored, and then Mom took over. Still, she lived a long life and died happy, as happy as any old dog could be when put to sleep.

And so will Mom. Not the being-put-to-sleep part. Is that even possible in New Jersey? No, I'm talking about the happy-about-dying-of-old-age part.

I love my mom. I do. But—forgive me for saying this. Forgive me for this even entering my mind—but there *is* a limit. This is why I chose not to have children. So, how patient do I need to be? I would greatly appreciate a hint. Any hint.

And just hearing my question, I realize you may be right. I don't have that "unconditional love" thing down. Not yet anyway. This parenting thing is so freakin' hard.

Okay. Be patient. I'll work on it. Really, I will.

Do me a favor? Let's keep this conversation between us, okay?

I love my job, I love my job, I love my job.

CHAPTER 50

Kleenex Tissues, Momma's New Best Friend

Mom sips her juice in bed.
I'm peeing at the same time.

—*Mom, my multitasker*

It seems that many, if not all, seniors are obsessed with Kleenex tissues. A Kleenex to stifle a runny nose, to catch a trickle of drool, or to erase, with a little spit, that smudge on a grandchild's face. Neatly folded or hastily balled, crammed up a sleeve or stashed in a pocket, cherished in any condition, and always at the ready, Kleenex tissues are a senior's best friend.

Mom also loved her Kleenex, perhaps more

than most. She used one tissue over and over until rendering it utterly useless. After each assault, she stuffed those soggy shreds up her sleeve for safe keeping.

When I first discovered this nasty habit and attempted to replace the old, tattered tissue with a new one, she immediately and unequivocally rejected my offer. When I tried to wrestle it from her clutches, she fought me tooth and nail. Extracting that trace of a tissue turned into a fierce battle of wills, more agonizing than separating an obstinate child from her baby blanket.

Was I battling the last bastion of the Great Depression? Did this pathetic clump of fibers represent something more than I realized? The answer was a resounding *no*. That brave tissue served her well. It lasted far beyond what the inventors intended or dared to imagine, and it deserved a swift and proper burial.

Mom may have been as stubborn as they come—and, at times, impossible—but she met her match with me. And I had no intention of giving in. Instead, I used my well-honed powers of persuasion I often employed during our time together.

"I'll give you this brand-new, right-out-of-the-box, super-soft tissue, good for several uses, in exchange for that disgusting, disease-carrying one." If she hedged, I added, "And the new one comes with a hot cup of tea."

Mission accomplished.

Hoping to avoid our own highly inevitable Kleenex addiction, my sister Laurel and I entered a pact. If either of us ever caught the other stuffing a tissue in any condition up his or her sleeve, they shall be put to death with the offender's blessing. So far, so good.

CHAPTER 51

House Calls? Who Still Makes House Calls?

Mom: Okay, I'll just say so long now.
Me: Where are you going?
Mom: I'm going home.
Me: You are home.
Mom: Oh yeah.

The last time a doctor made a house call to 247 Emmett Place, other than Mom's podiatrist, was after an incident in church in 1972. A spasm of vertigo had spun Mom back into the pew.

"I think I need to go home," she whispered.

I knew it must be serious because she never left Mass early. I helped her to her feet and gingerly escorted her down the main aisle. Every eye in the church focused on our every step. I wasn't sure if it was curiosity, concern, or condemnation. I only knew that it embarrassed me. Why would a fifteen-year-old helping his sick mother feel that way? I don't know. Later, guilt erased any embarrassment when I understood the gravity of Mom's condition.

The doctor diagnosed it as a Transient Ischemic Attack (TIA). TIA is a brief episode of neurological dysfunction resulting from an interruption in the blood supply to the brain, sometimes a precursor of a stroke. Mom, being Mom, recovered quickly and remained incident-free until a major stroke in 1993.

In the 1930s, house calls had made up 40 percent of doctor's visits. By the 1980s, they'd dwindled to 1 percent.[2]

So, in January 2013, when the phone rang and a voice asked, "Would Genevieve like a doctor who makes house calls?" I was shocked.

Two years ago, Mom's previous doctor had given her up for dead. We were doing fine on

---

[2] Danielle, "The Golden Age of House Calls and Home Physicians Returns," MD At Home (blog), August 16, 2017, https://www.md-athome.com/blog/home-physicians.

our own. Other than Digoxin, Mom had been medication-free since February 2011. Her monthly over-the-phone-remote-monitoring pacemaker checkups—very convenient, by the way—showed no cause for concern. However, getting her to and from those rare but necessary appointments often did more harm than good. So, I jumped at the opportunity to have a doctor who came to us instead.

A few days later, that sweet, soft-spoken doctor introduced herself. Mom clicked with her right away. After her initial assessment confirmed that Mom was not only well cared for but in good shape for her age, I clicked with her as well.

Unlike the in-and-out doctor visits of today, she took her time and never rushed. As an added convenience, she arranged to have all exams, sample takings, and even x-rays performed in our home.

When the mood-enhancing Verilux Happy-Light couldn't keep up with Mom's bouts with depression, the good doctor prescribed a low dose of the antidepressant Zoloft. In the first few weeks, I saw no noticeable change.

Then one morning while serving Mom breakfast in bed, she asked, "Why are you so good to me?"

"Because you're my mom and I love you," I said.

"You're a good kid," she replied.

I smiled and pumped my fist. Finally, the meds had kicked in.

During a visit later in the year, the good doctor whispered to me, "I think your mother has Alzheimer's," and suggested that Mom take a series of cognitive tests.

Depression and strokes can contribute to memory disorders, and Mom suffered from both. Early in our journey, she had some memory issues. In addition to forgetting my name, she claimed all of her kids attended her alma mater, Sewanhaka High School—an hour and a half away by car—instead of Ridgewood High, just five minutes on foot. She insisted her mother, who'd died weeks before my parents' wedding, had helped raise all six of her children. She saw imaginary people in vivid detail on her ceiling and outside her bedroom window. However, with all my experience playing doctors on TV, none of that screamed Alzheimer's. Not to me.

After all, she remembered how to guilt trip, how to cheat at cards, and how to steal my ice cream.

But I yielded, and the good doctor proceeded with the tests. They included marking a specific time with the hands on a clock, repeating a short list of words, counting backward from one hundred by sevens, and various drawing tests. Except for the short-term memory test, I thought Mom did well. The doctor, however, felt confident the results confirmed her suspicions.

I bristled at the thought, and being a good son, I jumped to her defense.

"She's ninety-one. I'd have trouble with some of those tests," quickly following up with, "And no, I will not take any of them."

But the good doctor stood firm.

So, I turned to Mom and asked, "You don't have Alzheimer's, do you?"

With a look of bewilderment and a shrug of her shoulders, she said, "I don't remember."

Priceless.

CHAPTER 52

When Ya Comin' Home?

(Mom wakes me extra early.)
Mom: I just wanted to chat.
Me: About what?
Mom: I have no idea.
(She falls back to sleep.)

I was fifteen the first time I stayed out all night. My best friend and I, competing for the same girl, slept on her porch just to be near her, and to keep an eye on each other.

In the morning I came home to find Mom sitting at the kitchen table. A sleepless combination of worry and anger weighed on her.

I apologized but explained as an ignorant teenager, "Don't worry. I can take care of myself."

This would not be the last time my actions caused her concern or prompted her to wonder or to ask, "When ya comin' home?"

Caring for Mom was more than a full-time job, but I also had another one: keeping Dad's dream alive. Grandpa Po's Originals had fallen on hard times after losing national distribution and much of our sales force. Michael and I struggled to keep the business afloat. He serviced his stores on the East Coast; I serviced mine out west. I also handled all online sales. I also produced every crunchy golden nugget. That meant I needed to return to my Los Angeles factory for a week every few months and crank my one-man operation into high gear. Working crazy hours, I prepped, cooked, seasoned, mixed, packed, palletized, and shipped three months' worth of Grandpa Po's Originals all in seven days. I called it Hell Week, and for good reason.

Laurel, who lived in Southern California, flew in to take over Mom's care during those weeks. She was a dutiful daughter but admitted one week was her limit before she'd blow her top dealing with Mom. For her, it was also Hell Week.

When I first broke the news about leaving, Mom batted her sad puppy-dog eyes and asked, "When ya comin' home?"

This became her constant refrain whenever I headed west.

When I called to check in, the first thing out of her mouth was, "When ya comin' home?"

When we FaceTimed, those doleful eyes filled my computer screen as she pleaded, "When ya comin' home?"

After swallowing my guilt, I offered my usual response. "As soon as I can, Mom. As soon as I can."

That seemed to pacify her, at least for the moment.

"When ya comin' home?" was a lovely affirmation to me, but I felt terrible for Laurel, who stood by Mom's side for many of those calls. It reminded me of the elderly lady at Senior Connections who had boasted about her sons while ignoring the daughter who stood by her side. Mom always was and continued to be tougher on her girls.

One day, in an attempt to ease her separation anxiety, Michael and I performed a coast-to-coast musical event on FaceTime. I played the Beatles' "Blackbird" on my guitar in Los Angeles while he sang with Mom at his side in New Jersey. After much encouragement, Mom accompanied him on the chorus.

It was sad and sweet, and she seemed satisfied. But when Michael gave her a celebratory kiss on the cheek, and I laid down my guitar, Mom batted her sad puppy-dog eyes and once again asked, "When ya comin' home?"

CHAPTER 53

Third Time, No Charm

Di-ver-tic-u-what? —Me

O nce in a while life throws you a curveball. On June 4, 2013, it threw me a humdinger.

It all started back in February at my annual check-up in Los Angeles. I was physically fit. I exercised daily. I ate a healthy diet. But my doctor said, "You're in your fifties. Get a colonoscopy just to be safe."

When I got back to New Jersey, I contacted Anthem for gas-troenterologists in my network and scheduled an appointment.

I researched the cost. The average price of a colonoscopy was $1,185. Having a high deductible, I expected to pay most of it, if not all. Curiosity got the best of me, so I called the doctor's office for a quote.

The nurse refused, stating, "Every case is unique."

This made me suspicious, but when she threatened me with a $200 cancelation fee I kept the appointment, trusting Anthem to protect me.

All appeared to go well. The doctor found and removed a benign polyp, and I felt no pain until the $8,500 bill arrived. Never trust your insurance company, but that's another story.

Feeling violated all over again, I canceled the $500 post-procedure appointment. The doctor retaliated by refusing to give me my full report. That report contained information that could have saved me a lot of pain physically, emotionally, and financially. So much for "do no harm."

Six weeks later, I felt a pain in my lower abdomen after working out in the gym in the renovated basement. Figuring I overdid it, I took a break the next day but returned to the gym the day after. That night, the pain got worse.

I checked out the symptoms on WebMD. *A hernia?* I had an umbilical hernia years ago. This felt similar. With proper rest, I hoped it would heal on its own.

Then on Tuesday, June 4, 2013, I was minding my own business while doing my business on the commode when *boom!*—an intense stabbing pain shook me to my core.

That night Michael cooked and cared for Mom. Good thing because I was in no condition to do so. I had chills, and even though it was ninety degrees with 90 percent humidity outside, I slept in flannel pajamas with a space heater running at full throttle. The fever broke and the pain subsided, but twenty-four hours later it returned with a vengeance. This was one hell of a hernia, but I continued to believe in healing thyself. So, I waited it out another day. Clearly, I didn't have my much-needed mother's intuition.

Finally, after doubling over again on Friday, I gave in and drove myself to the Valley Hospital emergency room.

"I have a pain in my lower left abdomen," I blurted out.

"Sounds like diverticulitis," the nurse shot back immediately.

"Di-ver-tic-u-what?" I'd never heard of it, couldn't even pronounce it, but they could. I was admitted after a doctor and a CT scan confirmed the nurse's initial diagnosis.

I called Michael.

"I'm in the hospital. It may be serious. You need to get someone to cover for me."

All I heard was, "Oh shit," not knowing if this was in response to his predicament or mine. Either way, "oh shit" summed it up.

The doctor also discovered a rupture in my colon, which had caused a life-threatening infection, which had caused my fevers. He didn't share the "life threatening" part with me until I was out of the woods, but he did share three scenarios to ponder.

1. Treat the infection with antibiotics. No surgery required.

2. Primary bowel resection. Traditional surgery to remove the diseased or ruptured part of the intestine, which is then reconnected to the healthy segment of the colon.

3. Bowel resection with colostomy. If the parts cannot be reconnected, all waste would collect in an external bag.

I had my preference, but my body had its own.

Surgery.

When the doctor broke the news, tears flowed. I worried about Mom. I worried about my snack business. And I worried about the long recovery. At twenty-six, I had abdominal surgery to repair my umbilical hernia. It laid me up for several months. How long would it take me to recover at fifty-six?

But I had no choice and little time to worry. The doctor scheduled surgery for the next morning. Caryl drove up from the Jersey Shore for moral support, but when the surgeon described the procedure, she totally lost it.

I grabbed her hand. "Don't worry. I'll be fine. Now get out of here. You're depressing me."

They couldn't determine scenario two or three until I was under the knife, which left my pooping future uncertain. Three hours later, I woke up in recovery and immediately searched for the dreaded colostomy bag. I came up empty-handed.

I thought, *this might suck, but it could've been worse.*

Later that night, it got worse. Much worse. I have a high-pain threshold like Mom, but when the anesthesia wore off, I thought, *This is ridiculous.*

"Give me the Michael Jackson cocktail and put me out of my misery," I begged the nurse.

Desperate, she called my surgeon. After several failed attempts, he came up with an effective pain-reducing, mind-altering cocktail that, along with the excellent ice chips, nearly made the entire experience tolerable.

Nearly.

While I was stuck in the hospital, not knowing when or if I'd ever get out, the search for my temporary caregiver replacement began.

Marina, whom Michael had hired to care for one of his clients, became available after a perfectly timed passing. Marina needed the work, and we needed the help. Unlike many of his previous hires, my Brother Teresa hit a home run with Marina. She stepped right in and picked up where I left off but understood and accepted my intention to resume my duties when able.

Eight days after bidding *adieu* to eight inches of my colon, I returned home to an emotional homecoming, but only in my dreams. No one told Mom where I'd been or that I'd almost died.

When I entered the kitchen, I felt like a ghost. Mom sat at the table eating her coffee ice cream with Marina by her side. Nothing could steal Mom's attention from that bowl of frozen delight. I was in too much physical pain to deal with that emotional punch to my stapled gut.

I hugged my mother and headed to the basement with my bounty of medications to begin my recovery. Just like at Valley Hospital, the well-equipped man cave provided all the necessities: an adjustable bed, a television, and a bathroom mere steps away.

I was in no physical condition to do otherwise, so I sat and observed Marina in action. Knowing I'd set a high bar, my siblings worried about how we'd get along.

Marina had a different way of doing things— no better or worse, just different. The critical issue for me was how she and Mom got along— all good on that front. Marina was a pro. She always dressed in white. She showed respect by addressing us as Miss Genevieve, Mr. Mark, and Mr. Mike. She needed no prompting, never left a mess, and even offered to care for me during my convalescence. *Nice.*

After sitting in silence for a few days, I added my two cents. Marina accepted only one. Ruffling my feathers was no way to start our working relationship, but seeing how serious she took her job, I yielded. And after seeing how serious I took mine, we bonded and became a formidable team. We shared the common goal of making Mom's life joyful and carefree.

But twelve days after my initial surgery, complications sent me back to the ER. A CT scan revealed an obstruction caused by adhesions which required me going under the knife again. This trip included a nurse jamming a nasal gastric tube—sans lubrication—up my nose and down to my stomach, a diet that consisted of ice chips for nine days, and the loss of twenty pounds I had no business losing. I also contracted MRSA, a deadly staph infection that required isolation or, in my case, semi-isolation with an obnoxious WWE wrestling fan who kept me up every night until 4:00 a.m. glued to the fake action on the TV.

After eighteen days of little sleep and little healing, my doctors released me back into the wonderful world where watching "professional" wrestling was still a choice.

By this point, Marina and Mom had their routine down, and it brought me greater relief than my bevy of painkillers.

Okay, maybe not.

Marina's years of practical experience did ease my concern. They came in handy when nagging issues persisted and when new ones emerged. She solved Mom's itching issue with a cream I'd never heard of. When the podiatrist had no solution for my mother's blood blister, Marina stepped in and healed it in days. And if Mom refused to eat, Marina spoon-fed her.

"Just one more, Miss Genevieve, just one more." And she didn't let up until the bowl was empty.

Marina, or as I called her, "My Savior from El Salvador," was always cheerful, kind, and patient. She also had an excellent sense of humor. And though nowhere near fluent in English, she got my jokes and often punctuated her hearty chuckle with, "Mister Marrrrrrk."

Even though she was devoted and tireless, Marina didn't treat herself well. She took Sundays off to go to church and stayed the night at her own apartment, and I assume, to sleep in a proper bed. But at our house, she curled up on the couch instead of sleeping on the futon bed I purchased for her.

Why? I don't know, but the first time I caught her we had a talk.

"I need you to be happy, healthy, and well-rested. So, please sleep in the bed."

She yielded.

With Marina well-rested and taking good care of Mom and me not content sitting still, I—perhaps sooner than recom-mended by four out of five doctors—returned to unfinished business: renovating the first-floor bathroom. Working late into the evenings, I often left the heavy lifting and cleanup for the next day. Every morning I'd wake up to find the workspace spotless, and all debris bagged and stowed in the garage. This workhorse of a woman possessed phenomenal strength and stamina. I guess she wanted to make sure I stayed happy, healthy, and well-rested too.

My Savior from El Salvador indeed.

After finishing Mom's house, I took on a new renovation project, for one of Michael's clients.

But in the spring of 2014, just as I regained

my strength and my twenty pounds, a familiar jab doubled me over again.

When my surgeon suggested I return to the ER, at first, I refused. "They never let me out."

He countered with a reasonable question. "What's the alternative?"

The third time was certainly no charm. Another CT scan revealed yet another obstruction, which required yet another surgery. This trip to the ER became a twenty-three-day hospital stay that included another NG tube—lubricated this time—another ice-chips-only diet, a new surgeon, the removal of three inches of my small intestine, the loss of my recently regained strength, and another twenty pounds.

I was not happy to be back in what now should be renamed, the Porro Wing. But I didn't take it out on the staff as I had witnessed so many patients do. I tried to have fun with them, even the dietitian who recited daily, and at full volume, the entire three-meal menu to my carousel of roommates while I endured my nine-day-ice-chips-only diet.

"Pamela, that's so unfair. They don't get ice chips?"

I made a special effort to be cheerful and to express my gratitude to all my nurses. Though it was not my intent, brightening their day paid big dividends, like foot massages, being a buffer between doctors with drill-sergeant bedside manners or coming to my rescue after my nine-day fast ended.

"All I want is a toasted English muffin with melted butter," I said.

"That's not on the menu," the dietitian insisted.

But a nurse overheard and smuggled in for me the Best Toasted English Muffin Ever.

"How do you take your protein?" another nurse asked me.

"That's a loaded question," I said. "I dare not ask you the same."

She cracked up and later helped move me to a private room for some much-needed peace and quiet.

Twenty-three days later I dragged my emaciated body, my even shorter digestive system, my long thrice-stapled incision surrounded by multiple laparoscopic ones, and my collection of painkillers home to begin my long, painful recovery all over again.

New Name, New Role

After my trio of surgeries, my nephew, Sawyer, gave me a new nickname: "Semi-Colon."

Funny, but I paid a painful price for that laugh. Also new was my caregiving role. Since I had a ticking time bomb that threatened to send me back to the ER at a moment's notice, Marina assumed full-time duties. Other than on her day off, I became a full-time observer.

There was a silver lining to my diverticulitis three-peat. It deepened my empathy for Mom, and it gave me a preview of what I could look forward to, hopefully, in the far distant future. I drank Ensure and Pro-Stat to keep up my strength, just like Mom. I required assistance on my daily walks, just like Mom. I had little control over my bowels, just like Mom. And as the powerful painkillers wore off, my skin got terribly itchy, requiring major scratching, just like Mom.

My experience also made me realize no one is immune to the physical and emotional stress of twenty-four-seven caregiving. Not even those in denial, like me. I ate well, I exercised regularly, didn't smoke, didn't drink too much.

Oh, I can handle this, I thought.

But lack of sleep was an issue, in addition to my constant worry. *Is Mom awake? Does she need anything? Is she still breathing?*

Not to mention the stress caused by months of dealing with Tammy and the Tweedles, renovating the house, struggling to keep my snack business alive, hosting holiday dinners, and generally wanting everything to be perfect. I didn't take proper breaks, in length or in number, because I wanted to keep my mother alive and happy. The irony of it all, she almost outlived me.

The pros know what they're talking about. My stress crept up and up and up until *boom!*

CHAPTER 54

Martini Anyone?

Mr. Martini, you have a hungry? —Marina

Alzheimer's rocked David and Kathy's world when it chose its next victim: Kathy's charming and elegant mother, Kay. And it wasted no time.

I always liked Kay. She was a no-nonsense woman, but ever the "sophisticated lady." Though painful to witness her steady decline, she and I managed to have some fun in its early stages. Whenever Kay had dropped by to visit Mom, it was always a surprise. A surprise for Kay, for us, and for the road she had no business driving on.

But I'd always greet her with a smile and ask, "Would you care for a drink?"

"A cosmopolitan would be lovely," she'd say without missing a beat.

While I prepared cocktails—sans alcohol, of course—Kay sat opposite Mom at the kitchen table. Since neither possessed the gift of gab anymore, their conversations had enough *Pinteresque* pauses to satisfy any theater enthusiast. And my virgin cosmos did little to loosen their tongues.

For Kathy's peace of mind and Kay's safety, she moved into an assisted-living facility. This left her Yorkshire terrier, Martini, needing a new home. Mom's love of dogs made the search short and sweet. However, the joy Martini brought Mom meant extra work for Marina and me. When this little guy got excited, as he often did, he peed anywhere and everywhere. Zuri redux?

A belly band—I called it a "dance belt" to protect his machismo—did little to curtail his excitement. So, I added a feminine pad. Machismo? To hell with that. I was tired of cleaning up the pee. Marina was too. Still, his belly bands needed washing daily. Good thing Martini was short and sweet, or he would have been in search of yet another home. *Rápido.*

It didn't take long for Martini to become Mom's new best friend. He soon became

Marina's too. The *très amigos* forged their bond watching *Pasión de Gavilanes*, a popular Spanish telenovela. Marina insisted Mom loved it, but I begged to differ. Every evening at eight o'clock, Marina, Martini, and Mom sat in the living room with their eyes glued to the television. And I guarantee you, two out of the three had no clue as to what was going on. After logging in all those hours of Spanish television, I feared Mom and Martini would only listen to me if I spoke, not only in Spanish, but in overly dramatic Spanish.

¡Ay, caramba!

CHAPTER 55

Halloween Delayed

*Mom: I don't have any idea how this place works—
the games, the house. How do I get credit?*

Me: You don't need credit. This is your house.

Halloween, both a strange and wonderful tradition, conjures up mostly fond memories for me. Strange because the night before—Cabbage Night to us in New Jersey, Mischief Night to others—we smashed pumpkins, toilet-papered trees, shave-creamed front doors, and egged everything in sight. And yet wonderful because the next evening we returned to those same houses, in disguise, said "trick or treat," and collected a sweet reward. Since we did no serious damage, we felt little guilt, if any.

As soon as the sun hit the horizon, we hit the streets. Armed with flashlights and pillowcases—no paper shopping bags could handle the loot we hoped to haul in—my brothers and I raced in opposite directions, gathering up goodies. We continued nonstop until the last house on the last street went dark. If anyone handed out a favorite treat, we'd make a quick costume change and return for a second helping. If our costume was a hit, people invited us in to get a better look. But who had time for chitchat? We had work to do.

At the end of the night, we dumped our loot on the living room floor to see who got the most. Michael, who was older and covered more ground, usually won. For diabetes, there were no losers. After the victory celebration ended, the trading began.

Twizzlers and Hershey bars with almonds were my favorites. A close second was Red Hots or Peanut M&M's. PayDay, Snickers, Baby Ruth, Goobers, Necco Wafers, Smarties, Sno-Caps, and SweeTarts were always good bargaining chips. The worst was raisins. Raisins on Halloween? What's wrong with people? They ranked down there at the bottom, along with candy corn and pennies. Nasty Mr. Tiegent—who put up a fence, blocking a public sidewalk so no one could venture near his house—always gave five pennies instead of a treat on the one day of the year he allowed us to grace his domain. We did so more out of curiosity to see what evil looked like up close, and we got our five cents' worth every Halloween.

One year, near the end of the night, a couple of lowlifes robbed Michael of his entire bounty, leaving him unharmed but devastated. We all pitched in candy to make up for his losses, though I can't guarantee any of my favorites made it into the charity bucket.

Mom loved Halloween. And why not? It gave her another excuse to shop. She also enjoyed greeting all the neighborhood ghosts, pirates, princesses, fairies, and superheroes. Instead of candy, she handed out sugar-free fare: potato chips, Cheetos, Fritos, and pretzels, but never the dreaded raisins.

My favorite costumes were Zorro and Frankenstein. But the cool-on-the-outside, hot-on-the-inside green rubber mask required too many breaks to mop the buckets of sweat that blurred my candy-seeking vision. So, Zorro became my go-to getup.

Those costumes came years after recovering from the psychological trauma inflicted on me by Mom. She dressed me up as the Madeline character, two years running. That costume must have been on sale, and Mom had no intention of letting it go to waste. And like Cinderella and the glass slipper—lucky me—I was the only one that *adorable* outfit fit. For those two Halloweens I did my best to disappear under that yellow hat, that curly red wig, and those scores of freckles. The giant yellow balloon almost made that costume worth it. *Almost.* That costume made me wonder if Mom really wanted a fourth girl instead of a third boy.

In high school, Halloween parties replaced trick-or-treating for most of us. Before heading out, I'd relieve Mom at the door of 247, sometimes dressed as Zorro. I greeted one kid with, "My costume's better than yours," and as he watched in horror, I dipped into his plastic pumpkin for my own treat. His mother, a few steps away, couldn't help but laugh. Before the kid totally lost it, I returned his candy, added a bag of chips, and sent him on his way.

Late one night, a classmate, way too old for trick-or-treating, rang our bell dressed as

Superman. My "Really?" sent his sad superhero-ass away, embarrassed and empty-handed. Sorry, fake Superman, treats are for kids.

Halloween 2012 was going to be my first at 247 Emmett Place since 1975, and I'm sure the first for Mom in many years. I had thought it was time to surprise the neighbors and remind them just how much fun the Porros were. So, I went shopping—it's in my blood—and searched far and wide for costumes for the two of us. I settled on the ever-popular Kermit the Frog and Miss Piggy. But Superstorm Sandy had its own surprise and dealt the East Coast the ultimate trick. So, I mothballed the Muppets until the next year.

On October 31, 2013, Kermit and Miss Piggy made their 247 Emmett Place debut. Mom had a ball entertaining the local kids for hours. It turned out to be her last Halloween, but she went out with a bang and a Miss Piggy *hi-yah!* karate chop.

CHAPTER 56

A Surprise Letter from an Old Friend

Better hurry. Mom's waiting. —Me

Two major events happened one week apart in October 1981: my brother David's wedding and my grandmother's funeral. David's marriage is still going strong. Josephine made it to ninety-four. At the funeral, my aunt Claire, bubbling more than usual, peppered me with all kinds of questions about college, my new job, my old girlfriend.

"How do you know all this?" I asked.

"Your mother keeps me up to date on you kids," she said. "She's so proud of you all."

Aunt Claire, the precursor to Twitter, quickly shared all the news about the six of us with her three children. Though we did nothing out of the ordinary, the constant barrage about us no doubt caused some resentment with our cousins. Hopefully not too much.

Making our parents proud is something we all hope and strive for. Mom and Dad each set a good example. Besides obeying the Ten Commandments, I watched my father open doors for women, stand whenever one entered the room, and always allowed them to go first. When you clap, make sure people hear it. When you shake a hand, make it firm. He wasted nothing. He squeezed out the last drop of toothpaste. He invented Envelope Soap to utilize those remaining slivers. He even swept his breadcrumbs into his coffee. If someone made a mistake in his favor, he corrected them, much to the surprise of many waitresses.

One of his favorite prayers was Others, as in *think of others*. He always did. And to inspire others, my dad, who displayed little if any vanity, sprang for a vanity license plate emblazoned with the word "OTHERS" for his Volkswagen Bug.

My mother taught her sons to be gentlemen, to walk on the street-side of the sidewalk to protect the woman from splashing water, or worse; to be the first on and off an elevator to make sure it was safe for a woman to enter and exit. She showed us how to Q-Tip our ears, push back our cuticles, and keep our elbows clean and moisturized. We learned to care for all living things. I never witnessed any prejudice or bigotry from either of them.

We witnessed how they handled crises. They met them head-on. They dealt with their own with dignity and grit, and their kids' with grace and determination.

Over the years, I heard many compliments about my parents, but didn't realize their impact on others until a surprise letter arrived in 2013. David's high school sweetheart heard I'd moved back to Ridgewood to care for Mom. She emailed me and asked if she could send Mom a letter. Curious, I said sure.

"Do you remember David's high school girlfriend?" I asked.

Mom's eyes lit up. "Kathy," she whispered.

Of course she remembered Kathy, whom she hadn't seen or heard from in over forty years. Why? Because Kathy didn't wipe my mother's butt. Since I knew wiping butt causes amnesia, I took no offense. Not too much, anyway.

I emailed Kathy a photo of Mom in her wheelchair, staring out the front window. It's sad, and sweet, and could move anyone with a pulse to tears. I included a note:

"Better hurry. Mom's waiting."

"You're killing me," she replied.

A few days later, her letter arrived.

What prompted her to write was a 1976 letter from my father she recently rediscovered. Dad had often sent carbon-copied typewritten letters to us kids, but this was the first I learned that included David's high school girlfriend. I never knew how close she and my parents had been.

She thanked Mom for treating her like a daughter and how much she appreciated all the lunches and shopping trips. I guess after wearing us out, Kathy was the only one willing and able.

Mom beamed as I read the letter. It was great to see her smile, which was somewhat rare in those days. I knew my parents were pretty damn special. But knowing others felt the same after all these years made me appreciate them all the more.

CHAPTER 57

My Chick Magnet

A passing lady: She's adorable. How old is she?
Me: Ninety-one-and-a-half.
Lady: Aww.

During one of my Los Angeles trips a friend became more than a *friend*, and we began a long-distance relationship. Never having had one, I jumped at the opportunity for a new adventure. She was weary, having had a painful one in the past, but she was willing to try again. It worked, for a while. We'd get together whenever she visited her daughter in the east and during my Hell Weeks out west. But having a complicated relationship with her own mother, she couldn't understand why I was so committed to mine. Most applauded my mission, and some even thought of me as a saint. I didn't see it that way, but I appreciated their approval and embraced their encouragement. Lack of both from my California girl caused tension, and soon it was back to the single life for me.

"Hi, I'm single, fifty-five, and live with my mother," might interest my psychiatrist neighbor across the street, but it was not a great opening line on the dating scene.

However, with a little genuine ingenuity, I could make my new reality work in my favor. Mom was like a puppy, my puppy. Who can resist a single guy with a puppy? Better yet, who can resist a single guy with a puppy in a wheelchair? (Unless they have mother issues, see above.) And the cuter, the better. So, I dolled her up, pulled her hair back in a ponytail, or for crowd-pleasing bonus points, a braid. I applied bright-red lipstick to match her freshly painted bright-red nails. I dressed her in her favorite pink outfit or—weather permitting—her eye-catching black ensemble with embroidered jacket, and voilà. After I dolled myself up, it was time to take my chick magnet for a ride.

As we strolled up and down the streets of Ridgewood, I could feel its magnetic power working. We drew lots of smiles from the local ladies. Lots of stares too. A few even stopped to chat. Unfortunately, the ladies were more interested in my mom and my mission than they were in me. It was probably best since Mom never approved of any of my previous girlfriends. I'd like to think she didn't think any of them were good enough, but who knows? In any case, she'd never accept a new one now. So, love had to wait. Anyway, it was getting late, and it was time to change my chick magnet's diaper and put her to bed.

CHAPTER 58

Three More Birthdays

Happy birthday to me.
—Mom singing with us.

W hen the Porro kids were younger, on every birthday we could count on clothes from Mom, a check from Dad, and cards from aunts Claire and Flo, who also always tucked in two crisp dollar bills. We could also count on impatient siblings rushing through the birthday song, praying for a quick wish and a swift blowing out of the candles so they could dig in to that Fishel's Bakery ice-cream cake. Other than that, the Porro celebrations were quiet family affairs. No big surprise parties for us. Though we had tempted fate twice, both nearly ended in disaster.

When Dad turned seventy and prepared for his new phase in life, we thought it would

be fun to celebrate with a surprise birthday/
retirement party at Caryl and Carl's home. We
lured our parents down to the Jersey Shore
under false pretenses. Family members who
came from near and far hid in the garage. As
Mom and Dad approached, Carl opened the
garage door and we shouted, "Surprise!"

Dad froze in his tracks, on the brink of a heart
attack, which froze many of us, on the brink of
our own. Fortunately, everyone survived.

We should have learned our lesson, but six
years later we planned a surprise party for our
mother's birthday/retirement. This time Mom
clutched her chest in shock. Our two surprise
parties nearly resulted in two of the shortest
retirements. So, no more surprise parties, at
least not for our parents.

A glutton for punishment, I took another
chance in 2000. Laurel survived her first fifty
years and Y2K, so I thought a special celebration
was in order. Since I knew only a few of
Laurel's church and teaching friends, I asked
her roommate to help track down some others.

Mom flew in from New Jersey to join the fun.
We held it at my Los Angeles apartment with
my unobstructed view of the iconic Hollywood

Sign—inspiring and motivating for those still in show business, demoralizing and depressing for those who were not. Laurel had expected a quiet birthday dinner with just the two of us, but as soon as she entered everyone screamed, "Surprise!"

Everyone except for Mom. She surprised me by being nowhere in sight. Concerned, I went in search and found her on the floor on the other side of my bed. She had lain down to hide and couldn't get up—a sign of things to come. Laurel had a surprise for me as well. Many of the "friends" her roommate invited were from an old address book, who came more out of curiosity, a few of whom Laurel had hoped never to see again. But she put on a smile and made the best of it. Although we avoided even a trace of tragedy, that was the last surprise party for us.

Birthday #1:
January 27, 2012

Mom's ninetieth birthday had been an unexpected gift, so I wanted the entire family to join the celebration. We needed a large space, one away from the Tweedles. David and Kathy came to the rescue by offering their ballroom dance studio. I took no chances this time. This was to be a "No Surprise" party. I designed invitations featuring Mom in her pink night-dress with her pink nose gorging on pink sherbet. Her favorite restaurant, Boston Market, catered the event. I scheduled it on a Saturday to make traveling easier for the four generations attending.

And travel they did. To Mom's delight, over twenty family members packed the studio where she held court for several hours. We topped off the evening with a grand ice-cream cake, but no one rushed through the song, prayed for a quick wish, or a swift blowing out of the candles on this birthday. We took it nice and slow before digging in. However, that luscious ice-cream cake with its chocolate whipped-cream icing staring us in the face did our patience no favors.

Birthday #2:
January 27, 2013

When Mom had taken that first bubble bath in the new upstairs bathroom—the bubble bath that nearly killed her—I had snapped a photo of her before disaster struck. In the photo, she's immersed in bubbles, grinning from ear to ear, and having the time of her life. Since it didn't capture the last time of her life, I used that shot of her in her birthday suit for her ninety-first birthday invitation. We celebrated at home, Mom and her kids. A quiet family affair, just like old times. But as we sat at that dining room table where we'd all grown up, nostalgia overcame us. The memories rushed in, the stories poured out, and the quiet disappeared.

"Do you remember pillow races?"

"How many times did you raid Dad's money sock?"

"Those plastic seat covers."

"The VW bug."

"That had plastic seat covers too."

On and on it went. Dad said he was always amazed by how well his children got along, how we truly enjoyed each other's company. It was something he and his siblings never experienced. The love in that room and the joy in Mom's heart filled me with pride.

Birthday #3: January 27, 2014

With her energy on the wane, I sensed Mom's ninety-second birthday would be her last. All six of her children were present, five in the room and Laurel via FaceTime. A few of her grandchildren and great-grandchildren also joined the celebration. Mom spoke few words but still managed to smile, blow out the candles, and finish the birthday song, ever so softly. When Caryl surprised her with a new stuffed doggy, it was love at first squeeze. Even though a somber cloud hung over this birthday, I cherished it as much as the previous two. And I will hold on to the memories of all three as tightly as Mom held on to her new stuffed doggy.

CHAPTER 59

The End Is Near

(Mom wakes with a furrowed brow.)

Mom: Take off my earrings so I can save them.

Me: For what?

Mom: When I die.

Me: Don't you want to wear them in Heaven?

*Mom: Yes, but I want them off now,
so I can save them.*

Me: You can keep them safe by keeping them on.
(She nods in agreement and falls back asleep.)

Mom only mentioned death to me in passing, as in our conversation about her earrings. More of a slip of the tongue than an icebreaker. Or perhaps it was me who wasn't ready for that talk. I knew she thought about it. Years ago, she floated the idea of cremation after the Catholic Church relaxed its restrictions on the practice. But other than her being buried next to Dad—an arrangement only agreed to three days before he died—and her expectation as a good Catholic to waltz through the pearly gates, we never discussed it in any depth.

She relished her busy social schedule of late, or so I thought. We had a well-attended traditional family dinner on Easter Sunday. Laurel came twice and even stayed beyond her seven-day limit. Michael continued his routine shifts. Caryl drove up from the Jersey Shore often to deliver her homemade cooking and handmade gifts. David came by more in the daytime than his usual late-night visits. Deecy and Big Mike made the fourteen-hour journey with their crew in the spring and again in the summer. Deecy's son, Owen, took a break from college to serenade Grandma Zennie on his cello. And several other grandchildren stopped by to say hello and to introduce their new additions. She loved seeing her grandchildren, and especially her great-grandchildren. At that point, she related best with the babies, a fellowship of the diaper brigade, I guess. Also, neighbors Ed,

Barbara, and Betty with her Welsh Corgi visited more often, much to Mom's delight. But now the joy seemed all but gone.

Something happened at 247 Emmett Place while I was in Los Angeles cranking out Grandpa Po's Originals. My latest trip required two Hell Weeks instead of my usual one, making it, other than my adventures in Valley Hospital, the longest time apart from Mom. When I returned, she spoke no words, barely smiled, and offered only a pitiful wave as Marina, looking less than her usual cheery self, pressed on with her spoon-feeding. "Just one more, Miss Genevieve, just one more."

The only spark of life appeared to be in Mom's right foot, as it tapped to a song no one else heard. Perhaps a heavenly choir calling for a new member?

Mom's diminished spirit not only saddened me but racked me with guilt. Was her busy social schedule too much? Did I stay away too long? Did my health issues contribute to her decline? Did my stepping in three years ago only prolong her misery? Would God speak to her again? Or did He already?

The change came so suddenly, and she so willing to sur-render to it. Dad hadn't wanted to die. He'd fought long and hard until his last breath.

"I have so much to live for," he'd said a few days before he passed.

And he did. He still had things he wanted to accomplish. His mind was sharp, but his body could no longer withstand the ravages of that damn heart disease.

Mom was not suffering, at least not physically. She just lost all interest in living, like before, except for that right foot tapping away to a mysterious song. The lone soldier still willing to put up a fight.

What caused this change? I needed to know. If for nothing else, to help me sleep at night. While bathing her on Marina's day off, I discovered the root. Mom loved her long locks. I did too. I spent a good part of three years washing and brushing it, and putting it into a bun, a ponytail, and braiding that beautiful white mane of hers. I once asked if she'd like to donate a portion to Locks of Love, a charity that made wigs for cancer patients.

"No, I don't want to," she said without hesitation.

I never revisited the topic, knowing she'd object to even the slightest of trims. But in my absence, someone had chopped off six inches.

This was not the first hair controversy at 247. During David's first year at college, he'd let his hair grow. By the time he returned home for summer break, it had reached past his shoulders. Dad didn't like the "hippie hair" and insisted, "Cut it or else."

David refused. When Dad promised to attack it with scissors while he slept, David called his bluff. Dad, however, made good on his threat. One afternoon, while his target napped in the living room, Dad went to town on the long brown locks with a pair of thinning scissors. I woke up with clumps of hair scattered around me. Dad's rage must have blinded him because, though David and I were similar in stature, I had much shorter hair. I marched into my father's room and pleaded my case. But taking no chances, I begged David to cut his hair, for my sake. He did, and from that day forward, I, too, kept my hair at my dad's approved length.

Was my father's kill-two-birds-with-one-stone move a mistake or genius? I'm not saying.

Like Samson, Mom's long hair seemed to be the source of her strength and vitality. It appeared a Delilah lurked in the shadows, waiting for the opportune moment to strike. Though Mom remained silent, Marina confided in me who had done the deed, but as we say in Porro Land, "Mum's the word."

I never asked why. What's done was done. Mom's precious long hair was gone. I feared our Battle of the Dutch Door was over and that the end was near, so I focused my energy on what lay ahead.

CHAPTER 60

Letting Go

*With what strife and pains we come into
the world we know not; but 'tis commonly
no easy matter to get out of it.*

—Sir Thomas Browne, Religio Medici, 1643[3]

Goodbyes have never been easy for me. It doesn't matter whether I'm too sensitive or emotional. I just don't like them. But they are, in most cases, unavoidable.

When I left for college, saying goodbye to my parents was hard, but my father's sense of humor made it easier.

"Want me to call to let you know I arrived safely?" I asked him.

"No, call me if you don't," he responded with a smile.

[3] Thomas Browne, *Religio Medici* (Frankfurt am Main, Germany: Outlook Verlag, 2019), 106.

When I left Ohio for California in 1984, saying goodbye to my two sisters was even more difficult. The three of us had graduated from The Ohio State University. We remained in Columbus many years after and grew especially close. Dad joined us for our "last supper" at a Greek restaurant. He flew out to help pack my car. That was my dad. Totally unnecessary but welcomed all the same. He could fit more in less space than anyone on the planet.

In between dinner courses, a violinist floated from table to table playing requested songs. Upon hearing of my move, he broke into "Sentimental Journey," and the floodgates opened. I offered him five bucks to stop and go away, and away he went.

Of course, all my previous goodbyes paled compared to my final goodbye to my father. It hurts still. In his last moments, I noticed how much he resembled his mother, which prompted me to say, "Say hi to Grandma for me." And he then took his last breath.

Or so I thought.

While on the phone with hospice, he gasped a few more times, making our final goodbye not so final. Which made me laugh, but it also made our *final* final goodbye all the more difficult.

My college girlfriend, Vicki, and her mother had dealt with their goodbyes in a unique way. When she visited home on weekends, they agreed that Vicki would wait until Monday for her mother to go shopping before packing her bags and heading back to college. No goodbyes, no shared tears, no never-ending hugs. Thank God my shopaholic mother had never thought of that. If she had, there's a good chance we would have never seen her again.

But for *this* goodbye, there would be no shopping for Mom, and no walking away for me. We were in this together. We'd been rehearsing for three and a half years. At one point in 2011, Mom had stopped breathing for a bit too long. I thought that was it. I swallowed my emotions and summoned the courage to say, "Mom, it's okay. You can go. We'll be fine."

But it wasn't her time. And yet, while doing my best to keep her alive and happy, the thought of that inevitable last goodbye lingered.

Throughout July and well into August, Mom retreated further into her silent, remote world.

This time, unlike three and a half years ago, her mind, body, and spirit were all in sync. No pumpkin pie would snap her out of it, nor umpteen bowls of sherbet. God would not intervene and tell her to "be patient." She'd been plenty patient. We all were. She, once again, was ready to go gently into that good night. And we, once again, prepared ourselves to say goodbye.

But while the rest of Mom's body slowly shut down, her right foot continued to tap to that mysterious song. As sad as we were, that bouncing foot made Marina and I laugh. Perhaps its purpose all along.

In between bounces, Catholic Daughters of America called. Mom was a longtime member of this Order, which supported the Catholic Church, the clergy, and various educational and charitable causes.

Catholic Daughters: I'm calling to let Genevieve know that her membership is expiring.

Me: There's no need to renew. She's close to expiring herself.

Catholic Daughters: Oh. Well, that's why we're here.

Me: She almost died three years ago. Where were you then?

Catholic Daughters: We didn't know.

Me: A priest delivered the Last Rites, and you didn't know?

Catholic Daughters: That's why continuing her membership is important.

Me: Are you saying if she doesn't pay, you will not be there for her this time?

Catholic Daughters: I didn't say that.

Me: Sounds like you did.

By the way, the only Catholic daughters who showed up at the funeral were Mom's own.

The dance with death is no fun, for the dancer or their loved ones. My dad went quickly. He was active, lucid, and he danced until his last day. It had been weeks since Mom showed any interest in dancing. And while she appeared to be in a rush to stop living, she was in no hurry to die. But I promised myself I'd stay with her—as I did with my father—until she took her last breath, no matter how long that took.

Tuesday

Mom had trouble chewing and swallowing. She vomited at 3:00 p.m. after drinking Gatorade—there goes that endorsement. She tried a piece of corn cake at 6:00 p.m., only to vomit again. We stopped all solid foods and most liquids. In the evening she felt a slight pain for the first time. I discovered a bulge in her belly. Possible hernia? From what, I'm not sure. Then her upper dentures dropped, causing breathing issues. I removed, cleaned, and placed them on the night tray in case she insisted, as usual, on wearing them to bed. She did not. Also, a first. I sensed we'd started the final countdown.

"I'm taking over," I told Marina. "I'll call you when I need you."

She understood and retreated.

After texting updates to my siblings, nieces, and nephews, I sat in Mom's wheelchair, stuffed a pillow under my chin to keep my head propped up, cradled her warm hand in mine, and began my vigil.

"I'm here, Momma, I'm here," I whispered.

She squeezed back and held tight.

During our journey, Mom always responded to touch. Some of my favorite moments were when we sat at the kitchen table holding hands in silence. But knowing that hearing was the last sense to go, I talked to her throughout the night, perhaps more for my comfort than hers.

Wednesday

Marina relieved me at 5:00 a.m. I tried to break away, but Mom held on.

"I'm just going to lie down for a bit," I whispered. "I'll be back soon."

She reluctantly released my hand. I got some sleep while Marina bathed and dressed her.

A few short hours later, I awoke to crying coming from Mom's bedroom. Fearing the worst, I sprang from my bed in a panic and stumbled down the stairs to find Caryl sitting with her. Mom was still with us. I took a deep breath and relaxed. I stood in the hall and listened in as Caryl told Mom how much she loved her and how exciting heaven would be, and that she would soon see all the people she had lost: our dad, her mother and father, her baby sister, her aunts Jo and May, and her uncle

William. Mom's eyes remained vacant. Caryl left the house an emotional mess. She never returned until the funeral.

Mom's difficulties continued, first with liquids, then breathing, and then when a disturbing gurgling began. Concerned, I contacted her doctor. She said it was time for hospice. They arrived the next day.

Thursday

I held Mom's hand until 6:00 a.m. We had brief moments when we'd connect, when I'd catch a twinkle in her eye. Those moments soon faded, but each morning it got more difficult to free my hand from hers.

"Momma, I just need to take a nap," I whispered. "I'll be back soon."

Marina filled in while I crashed upstairs.

A hospice nurse arrived to perform her initial exam. Michael and I shared power of attorney, but since I was present—physically, not mentally—I was tasked with signing a new do-not-resuscitate order. This was all too real now. There would be no more interventions.

No more doctors. No more emergency medical services. Mom would receive only end-of-life care. Although this was her wish, the weight of signing that document caused me to pause and take a deep breath before I put pen to paper. Still, my hand trembled.

Throughout the day, Mom drifted in and out of conscious-ness. She opened her eyes only on occasion, and though they remained vacant, she continued to respond to sound and touch. I downloaded some soothing Irish music for my Irish mother and played it day and night. "You Raise Me Up" by the Celtic Women makes me cry to this day.

Her grandson Abe visited and sat opposite me and held Mom's right hand. She squeezed her appreciation. Abe and I reminisced for a few hours before he crashed in the guest room. I stayed with her until seven the next morning. Only after once again pleading with Mom to release my hand, I got a much-needed few hours of sleep. With her near-death grip gaining strength, I feared I might never escape the actual one.

Friday

Hospice delivered the familiar white box of comfort, first introduced to me three and a half years ago. It contained various drugs to manage pain, anxiety, fever, etc. None were needed back then, but I believed much of it would be this time.

Mom felt a sharp pain in her stomach during what would be her last stop on the commode. When I asked if she wanted medicine, she nodded yes. With her high-pain threshold, I knew it was serious. I ran to the kitchen to get the morphine, but before squirting a full dose under her tongue, I sampled it on mine. Horrible stuff. Now I know why people prefer the needle. Fortunately for Mom, her taste buds were pretty much out of commission, so she had no problem with it. It worked fast. The pain subsided. However, it returned in the afternoon, requiring another dose. I put aside a dose or two for my own comfort.

The previous nights had been hell on my back, so I moved the red recliner next to Mom's bed. That's where I slept the next few nights. Abe visited again. We held Mom's hands throughout the night. She squeezed tight, not wanting to let go. Abe and I joked about her surprising strength.

At 4:00 a.m., Deecy, Big Mike, and two of their sons, Connor, and Sawyer, arrived from Michigan.

Saturday

Mom felt pain again in the morning. I administered another dose of morphine. At this rate, my stash was no longer safe.

Later I offered her a Popsicle—always one of my favorite treats. She nodded yes. I held it while she sucked. The cold liquid made her smile.

David dropped by in the afternoon. I suggested it might be time for the Last Rites again. He made the call.

"She's going soon," I added. "I think you should spend more time here."

Mom lay unconscious when the doorbell rang, but as soon as the young priest crossed the bedroom threshold, her eyes snapped open, she flashed a broad smile, and spoke for the first time in weeks. "Hello."

He was taken aback, having been told she was on her deathbed. "Hello, Mrs. Porro."

Also taken aback, I glared at her and said, "If you stand up, I'll kill you myself."

The priest chuckled.

Mom all but ignored me and kept her eyes locked on the Man of the Cloth. Once a Catholic, always a Catholic. But I have to say, he delivered a compassionate Last Rites, far different from the previous Last Rites phoned in by an apathetic priest three and a half years ago. And as soon as he left, Mom's moment of consciousness ended, and she fell back asleep.

David returned that night. We sat in the dark, on opposite sides of the bed, holding Mom's hands. We said little to each other. We used to be so close. Though two and a half years apart, people always thought we were twins. We both had worked at the local Dairy Queen. We'd hung out in high school. Vacationed together. When we'd hosted parties, we didn't serve the usual pretzels and chips. Instead, David insisted we treat our friends to hand-carved roasted turkey and hors d'oeuvres, which made our soirees the talk of the town. I watched with pride as he won his first schoolyard fight in our first year in public school. I cried the night a puck nearly blinded him at a hockey game. I was best man at his wedding. When he froze while buttoning his dress shirt and asked, "What am I doing?" I snapped him out of it. I had always admired how he used his ballroom dance skills to make any partner float like Ginger Rogers. He's still one of the funniest people I know.

But over the years a chasm grew between us. I'm not sure when it began, or why. Maybe he never got over me getting the better costume at my Lincoln Center debut, or my taking the best piece of meat on steak night. I grew to be the tallest of the boys. Maybe that was it. But I never held a grudge for the years of torture he inflicted on me. It toughened me up. Religion, politics? No doubt. Maybe my threatening him that one afternoon played a part. He had a nasty temper as a teenager. During an argument with Mom, he'd slapped her. Stunned, she just turned and walked away.

I stepped in and said, "If you ever raise your hand to her again, I'll kill you."

Fortunately for us both, he never did.

Whatever the reason for our rift, it's a shame, and sitting in the dark, opposite my brother whom I'd lost long ago only magnified the heartbreak of losing my mom.

Sunday

Much to my surprise, she woke up in the morning.

"Can I get you anything?" I asked.

Her eyes lit up.

"Coffee ice cream?" I offered, knowing it was her favorite.

She nodded ever so slightly.

I ran to the kitchen. While I dished it out, Marina mixed in some Digoxin, hoping it would help. I sat Mom up and spoon-fed her. She savored only a few bites before passing out again.

Later, while washing her face, she opened her eyes again for just a moment. She mouthed a silent, "I love you."

I kissed her forehead. "I love you too, Momma." I took a deep breath and once again summoned the courage to say, "You can go whenever you want. We'll be fine."

Those silent words were her last.

In the afternoon, the fish-out-of-water breathing began, and the gurgling became constant. This signaled the shutting down of her respiratory system. The stress on her face intensified. At one point she turned and shot a sinister look that rattled me—perhaps sending death a message. The final battle was underway. As recommended, I dispensed regular doses of morphine throughout the day.

A new hospice nurse came to replenish the kit. Deecy and I asked her about the gurgling.

"It disturbs the family more than the patient," she insisted.

I found this unacceptable and pressed her to please lessen it. Yielding, she attempted to extract the phlegm with a large syringe-like device I found more horrifying than the gurgling, and not at all effective. She gave up and ordered a secretion patch to appease me.

The nurse meant well, but this wasn't the first issue I had with hospice. In our first go-round, in addition to all the rebels, they'd delivered an enormous and cumbersome mechanical hoist to get Mom in and out of bed. She was not totally helpless, nor were we. We never used it, and hospice never removed it. Instead, it sat in the corner collecting dust for three and a half years. They also ordered an over-engineered wheelchair with extended head and leg supports. It would have been a good idea if it had any chance of fitting through the narrow doorway. The standard chair worked just fine for us.

After being absent for days, Michael appeared with a bottle of whiskey and a Q-Tip. Baffled, I watched him douse the cotton swab with whiskey and dab it on our unconscious mother's lips.

I jumped to stop him. "What are you doing? Whiskey and morphine don't go together."

He backed off, but only after completing his mission. He later told me he wanted to pay tribute to Mom, who had stayed up those many nights reviving our various pets with a drop of whiskey on their lips. A lovely gesture. One I would have championed if I'd only known ahead of time.

We all grieve in our own way.

Mom's gurgling grew louder and more disturbing. With no secretion patch in sight,

I rolled her on her side and let gravity do its magic. The steady stream of thick gray phlegm that flowed out shocked me. Sir Isaac Newton came through again, like he had with the Miracle Poop. I needed to introduce Sir Isaac to hospice.

Since the Porro-Newton technique continued to lessen the gurgling, I kept Mom on her side. When the mucus got too thick, I extracted it with the large sponge swabs from the hospice kit. I kept her lips and mouth moist with dabs of water. All of this might have been unnecessary, but it seemed to ease both Mom's anxiety and mine, so I pressed on.

In the late afternoon, Mom opened her eyes and she puckered up for a kiss, letting me know she was still here, she was still my momma, and she still loved her kisses. I cherished those moments, but regrettably, that was our last.

Her gasps grew weaker with each passing hour. Marina came in to check on us. She inspected Mom's feet and said, "She's ready." Then her emotions got the best of her, prompting a hasty retreat. I suspected she grew too close to yet another patient.

The pharmacy finally delivered the secretion patch at 8:00 p.m. I applied it, and it worked like a charm.

I had been up for the better part of five days. I was both physically and emotionally exhausted, but my mother was gasping her last breaths. I needed to stay awake. I needed to keep her tongue moist. I needed to keep talking to her. There was no time to register my heartbreak. That must wait.

Around 3:30 a.m., I shut my eyes just for a bit. When I opened them, I found Mom cold, clammy, and running a temperature. I must have dozed off. For how long I don't know, but now I was wide awake and in full panic mode.

"I'm so sorry, Mom. Please forgive me." I quickly applied cold compresses to bring her fever down. Then I remembered the hospice kit. My watery, bloodshot eyes struggled to read the directions for battling a fever. By some small miracle I managed. I rolled Mom onto her side, donned a sterile glove, and inserted a suppository. It worked fast. Her fever broke. I changed her diaper, nightgown, and the bedding, and then collapsed in the red recliner and prayed Mom didn't hear any of that drama. But if she did, I'm sure she got a kick out of it.

Big Mike checked in on us at 4:00 a.m.

"She's going soon," I whispered.

Deecy joined me soon after and stayed. The secretions had stopped but the cold sweats persisted. For the next couple of hours, I continued applying cold presses, holding her hand, talking, fighting to stay cheery. If she ever opened her eyes again, I wanted to make sure she saw a smiling face.

Monday, August 25, 2014

Shortly after 6:00 a.m., everything sped up. The stress and strain on her face intensified. Then I felt her hand go limp. Her fingers turned blue. The color drained from her face. When her gasps came fast and furious, I called hospice. They recommended Lorazepam to help relieve her anxiety.

"And what about mine?" I joked.

They didn't answer.

As the medicine kicked in, Mom's body relaxed. Her breaths grew weaker, the distance between them greater, until she took her last at 6:33 a.m. In that instant, a stillness fell over the room. The stress on her face melted away, as did many of her years. Her rosy complexion returned. For the first time in weeks, she looked at peace.

"Goodbye, Momma. Have a good trip. Say hi to Dad for us."

CHAPTER 61

Our Journey Comes to an End

Mom: I'm saying goodbye.
Me: Where are you going?
Mom: Heaven, I hope.
Me: Why?
Mom: Well, I'm not going to hell.
Me: Of course not, but why now? I just fixed up the house.
Don't you want to enjoy it? (No response.)
And I just bought three bags of crunchy granola.
(She laughs and falls back asleep.)

After kissing Mom on the forehead and wishing her a good trip, Deecy and I FaceTimed Laurel in California. She wanted to see Mom and say goodbye. I woke up

Marina. We hugged and cried, and I thanked her for all her help throughout the past year. Then I texted my nieces and nephews, "Grandma Zennie's in heaven."

Michael and David waited for the call no child wants to answer. When I broke the news to Caryl—as I did when Dad died—I asked, "Do you want to see her and say goodbye?"

"No, I said goodbye on Wednesday," she said. "I don't think I could handle another."

This came as a great relief.

Seventeen years earlier, when the funeral home had come for Dad, I refused to release him until everyone had a chance to say their goodbyes. Caryl lived ninety minutes away.

The attendants weren't happy, but I warned them. "Believe me, if you deny my sister this, it will not be pretty."

As she raced up the Garden State Parkway, the Porro kids thought it would be a good idea to surround our devoted Catholic father and recite the Rosary. Following Laurel's lead while Michael kept score on one of Dad's rosaries, we—all but one lapsed Catholics—stumbled through the Apostles' Creed, the Hail Marys, the Our Fathers, and the Glory Be's. Hearing us struggling with these traditional prayers that had been practically tattooed on our brains in parochial school surely would have sent Dad spinning in his grave. Lucky for us, he wasn't buried yet. Halfway through, Michael noticed a few of the Rosary beads felt odd. Upon inspection he discovered that Dad had replaced the missing ones with drops of hot glue. It was funny, sad, and at that very moment, perfect. Hot glue and duct tape were Dad's go-to solutions for repairing anything and everything.

An hour and a half later, Caryl burst through the front door. "Is he still here?" Before I could say yes, her pent-up emotion erupted in a primal scream that shook the house and everyone in it. It was raw, visceral, and to me, *beautiful.*

Later that night, Michael remarked about her scream. "Did you hear her? You would have thought somebody died," forgetting the events of the day.

I leaned in. "Somebody *did*."

He grasped the irony. "Oh, yeah."

We all grieve in our own way.

There would be no repeat of the Rosary challenge for Mom—a Catholic, but not as strict as Dad. Deecy and I stayed with her until the funeral home arrived. The only sound in the room was her pulsating air mattress. I should have turned it off earlier, but I just couldn't bring myself to do it. I wanted Mom to be as comfortable as possible for as long as possible. I know it made no sense, but sense would come later.

When two funeral home attendants arrived, they asked me to remove her necklace and earrings.

I knew how much she'd wanted to wear her earrings in heaven, so I asked, "Can we leave her earrings in?"

They nodded yes.

Then I handed them Zuri's ashes to be placed in the coffin per Mom's wishes, to which they also agreed. I left the room, necklace in hand, and didn't return until the funeral van drove away. I'd refused to see either of my parents in body bags. Both had died in peace, in their beds, at home with loved ones by their side. They both had exited this world the way most would envy. That's the image I chose to carry with me, not one of them in a bag.

The funeral home scheduled the Mass and Mom's burial for two days later.

"Why the rush?" I asked.

They reminded me that Mom had requested a natural burial—bravo—which meant no embalming, which meant getting her into the ground fast. No wake, no open casket, which I'm sure brought great relief to our funeral director who witnessed my moment of madness at Dad's wake back in 1997.

As I had slipped a photo from our Italy trip and some Nutra Nuts into my dad's pocket, I noticed something strange, something was off. I asked Deecy for a second opinion. She agreed. He was still handsome, but . . . then it clicked. The hair. They'd parted it on the wrong side. Dad always parted it on the left. We had given the funeral parlor a photo as a guide. How could they have gotten it so wrong? No way we were going to bury him like that. We needed to fix it and fix it fast before they opened the doors for the public viewing, just minutes away.

I tracked down the funeral director and asked him for a comb and hairspray. Aghast, he resisted, but I had *that* look. I won't say if it was crazed or not, but it was definitely one that said, *I'm grieving, and I mean business.* He returned with the requested items *pronto*.

As I leaned over the coffin, vying for the best angle to attack the problem, the funeral director backed away. When I hopped up and straddled it, he ran and shut the doors to shield the public. While family members watched in horror, I got to work. Feeling the need to explain, I whispered, "Sorry, Pop, I've got to fix your hair."

After a minute or two, along with Deecy's keen eye, we put our father back to his old self. Now he was ready to welcome family and friends fortunate enough to not witness my moment of madness.

We all grieve in our own way.

I have no regrets, and I'm sure it made Dad smile.

Shock comes in all forms, affects us in strange ways, and sometimes hits us when we least expect it. With Dad, it sprang. With Mom, I was still waiting. But I know this for certain. I was now without the two people who brought me into this world. I was fifty-seven years old, and I was an orphan.

The downside of living a long life is that few of your loved ones are still above ground, and fewer still are able to attend your final farewell. At ninety-two and a half, Mom had outlived her husband, all of her bridesmaids and their husbands, and most of her friends and relatives. Yet with all her children, grandchildren, great-grandchildren, spouses, and neighbors, the turnout, even on short notice, was pretty impressive. And the mood was more celebratory than sad.

Want to Hear a Joke?

Weeks before Mom's passing, Michael shared a joke with me. When I heard the punchline, I'd said, "Mom would be the only one to get that right."

Little did I know my comment would inspire Michael's eulogy. Amid a long Catholic Mass and thirteen minutes into his tribute where he skillfully weaved in Mom's proofreading prowess and stories of her caring for our sick pets, we were all more than ready for him to wrap it up. To everyone's surprise and to my delight, he closed with this:

Seventeen years ago, Dad died and went to heaven. Peter greeted him at the pearly gates.

Peter: Noel, you did a good job on Earth, but I have one more test for you before you can enter.

Dad: A test?

Peter: A spelling test.

Dad: I'm better at math.

Peter: Don't worry. It's easy. Spell "love."

Dad: Love? L-O-V-E.

Peter: Congratulations, you're in.

Years later, Peter retired, and Dad becomes heaven's gatekeeper. He takes great pride in administering the final test to those hoping to enter. One day, in the distance, he sees a familiar face approaching.

Dad: Genevieve, is that you?

Mom: Noel?

Dad: Wow, it's been a long time.

Mom: I tried to come sooner, but—

Dad: I know, "Be patient."

Mom: Was that you?

Dad: No, no.

Mom: Why are you out here?

Dad: I'm the gatekeeper.

Mom: Good for you.

Dad: So, before you can enter there's a little test.

Mom: A test?

Dad: A spelling test.

Mom: Really?

Dad:Don'tworry.It'seasy.Spell"Czechoslovakia."

Mom: (She narrows her eyes, then rattles off)
C-Z-E-C-H-O-S-L-O-V-A-K-I-A.
Dad: (grinning) On the ball, Gen. On the ball.

As Michael left the podium, the congregation broke into applause, quite unusual at a Catholic Mass. I whispered to myself, "On the ball, Mike. On the ball."

A Message from Heaven?

Before Deecy headed home, she took a stroll through the aisles of family items stored in the basement of Michael's offices. While searching for high school mementos, she came upon an old pencil box with a map of the world on its lid and a dial on the bottom. Turn the dial to choose a country and its capital appeared in the opposite window. No one had seen or touched this pencil box in decades. I never knew it existed, but I believe Mom did. The country displayed in the dusty window was "Czechoslovakia."

And its capital? Mum's the word.

Later that night, I sat alone in Mom's room on her red recliner. I stared at her empty bed and listened to the echoes of her last breaths. Only then did I finally let go and allowed my tears to flow. And boy, did they. I'm talking Old Testament. I was never one to shy away from tears, but this was ridiculous.

Our journey finally had come to an end. And through it all, through the thick and thin, the ups and downs, the trials and tribulations, I can honestly say, "I loved my job, I loved my job, I loved my job."

EPILOGUE

Mark's Vision

"Have a good trip. Say hi to Dad for us." —Me

I stand frozen in that surreal moment, staring at Mom. The pulsating air mattress continues to breathe, keeping her lifeless body afloat. I should turn it off, but I don't. The sound comforts me. Then a strange force compels me to look out her bedroom window. To my surprise, that parade of young children appeared. The parade Mom saw so often. All well-dressed and looking like they'd just escaped Mass at Our Lady of Mount Carmel. The girls in pigtails, ponytails, or pixie cuts wear frilly white dresses, white lace socks, and patent-leather shoes. Each carries flowers: single stem or bouquet. The boys with their combed hair, starched white shirts, dress pants, and shiny black shoes. They hold brightly colored balloons, just like Mom described.

As they round the cul-de-sac and pass by our house, the children wave to me. I wave back. But when I see the last child, I freeze and my heart jumps. It's the girl from the black-and-white photo on Mom's front wall. Eight-year-old Genevieve. She's dressed in the frilly white dress and patent-leather shoes, and holds a posy of daisies, but now she also wears Mom's earrings. The same earrings Mom wanted to wear in heaven.

The parade moves on, but young Genevieve lingers. She flashes me a familiar smile. I turn back to the bed. The stress on Mom's face has melted away, as have many of her years. Her rosy complexion is back. For the first time in weeks, she looks at peace. I turn back to the window. Young Genevieve is gone. The sidewalk is empty but for the posy of daisies.

"On the ball, Mom. On the ball."

Afterword

*As caregivers, one either becomes a better person
through compassion, patience, and humor,
or they become embittered and angry.*

—*Wendy Lustbader*[4]

At the time of this writing, it has been eight years since my mother passed. I now live in the South of France, in the village of Pézenas, in a sixteenth-century house on a cul-de-sac, second from the end on the right. I grew up in Northern Jersey, in the village of Ridgewood, in a much younger house but on a cul-de-sac, second from the end on the right. I didn't realize the coincidence until months after moving here, but how cool is that? When I first visited Pézenas, where they say Molière was born, I immediately felt at home, and after only five days there, I decided to make it my home. Perhaps my French ancestors spoke to me or

---

[4] Wendy Lustbader, *Counting on Kindness: The Dilemmas of Dependency* (New York: Free Press 1991).

instead spoke to the locals to make my move happen tout de suite. Or perhaps the wine had something to do with it. Anyway, it's a lovely place to live, a lovely place to reflect. Both have provided me the time and the motivation to write this memoir.

Tears kept me from finishing this book sooner. Emotions tend to rise quickly in me when it comes to family. Time does heal, but revisiting the events contained within challenged that adage and stalled the writing process for years. My notes, photos, and videos helped me capture and preserve those precious, funny, poignant moments that surely would have been lost.

Fortunately, through my journey with Mom I became not embittered and angry, but a better person, a better son, a better sibling, and a better friend, though some may disagree.

Mom could be a handful. When she descended deep into melancholy or appeared cold and unappreciative—making a difficult job even more difficult—I maintained my focus and never wavered from my goal to make her last years the envy of others. Compassion, patience, and the indispensable sense of humor came into play daily and often all at once. Although

I expected little in the form of gratitude from Mom, I got plenty. A smile, a squeeze of my hand, or her puckering up for a kiss was all I needed. If she added a chuckle, all the better. Those intimate gestures signaled I was on the right track.

Both Mom and Dad—if I may say—had good end-of-life experiences. They suffered little pain, died at home, in their beds, accompanied by loved ones. Though ever-present in my thoughts, I miss them terribly. I miss their phone calls. I miss their wit and humor. I miss Dad's letters and Mom's beautiful handwriting. I miss seeing them at opposite ends of the table at Thanksgiving, Christmas, and Easter dinners, leading us in prayer. I miss the sound of Mom and our dog, Gina, snoring in the afternoons (only one worked the graveyard shift). I miss Dad's well-worn jokes, his funny-shaped pancakes, and the aroma of instant coffee wafting through the house on weekend mornings. I miss Mom's "doohickies," "thinga-majigs," and "whojamacallitwhatsits" when she forgot what she was searching for. I miss Dad's "whoops" when he farted. I miss running my fingers through the cool satin edge of my parents' blanket. I miss Dad sharing his pink hand cream at night, soothing his sore hands, and keeping ours soft. I miss Mom's earlobe nibbles and Eskimo kisses. I miss the smell of my father's wallet. *Don't ask.* I miss trips to Grandma's house and her parting gift of a twist-tied baggy of licorice treats that rarely survived the drive home. I miss rub-a-dubs, Dad's fun way of bouncing us on his knees while toweling us off that always made us look forward to our evening baths. I miss our family reunions in the 1990s that no longer took place without our nucleus, our glue. I could go on, but you get my point.

I take comfort in knowing that I stepped up in Mom and Dad's time of need, left nothing unsaid, and stayed with them until each took their final breath. I take pride in having rebuilt 247 Emmett Place for a new family to move in and create their lifetime of memories on a cul-de-sac, in the second house from the end on the right.

References

Browne, Thomas. *Religio Medici*. Frankfurt am Main, Germany: Outlook Verlag, 2019.

Danielle. "The Golden Age of House Calls and Home Physicians Returns." *MD At Home* (blog). August 16, 2017. https://www.md-athome.com/blog/home-physicians.

Lustbader, Wendy. *Counting on Kindness: The Dilemmas of Dependency*. New York: Free Press, 1991.

Sparks, Nicholas. *The Wedding*. New York: Grand Central Publishing, 2003.

Vandiver, Willard D. Speech. 1899. US Navy Yard, Philadelphia.

Acknowledgments

I've always enjoyed memorializing family events: poems summing up our summer family reunions, memory books marking momentous occasions, *Ciao Celle*, my documentary of Dad's odyssey in Italy. *A Cup of Tea on the Commode* represents my latest effort. My siblings and others contained within will no doubt have different recollections of shared events, or object to revelations previously unknown. But this is my story, my journey. I've tried to be fair and honest. We all have faults. Many of mine pepper these pages.

Perhaps in hoping to evoke feelings of nostalgia, I've revealed too much. Nostalgia is a funny word. In Greek, *nostos* means "return home" and *algos* means "pain." Returning home can be painful, but good can come from it. Healing can come from it. That is my wish.

I want to thank Mom and Dad, the original multitaskers. You set the wheels in motion. I hope I didn't drive too far off the road in my attempt to honor you. For a few I'm sure I did, and then some. Thank you to my brothers and sisters for their love, trust, and support. And a special shout-out to Michael, the guardian of Mom's finances. Your diligent work on that end allowed me to do my diligent work on Mom's. Thanks to my nieces, nephews, grandnieces, and grandnephews, who always made Mom smile. Thanks to our neighbors Ed, Barbara, Irma, Betty, and Scottie. Your visits meant a lot. To the hospice nurses and aides who shared their knowledge, experience, and common sense, I thank you. Thanks to Marina and Martini, you brought comfort to us both. I'd also like to thank Tammy and the Tweedles, who made this journey a certainty.

A big thank you to my WriteLife Publishing team. You said yes to a new writer who didn't possess any of the trendy, easy-sell qualities that could guarantee his first book would be a trendy, easy-sell success. Special thanks to my editors, Andrea and Allison for your clarity.

And to Marybeth, Kathy, Lisa, and Maura, my Our Lady of Mount Carmel crushes who always ignored me when Mrs. Ryan made me demonstrate ballet positions in front of our third-grade class. I now live in the South of France, and with none of you. Oh, and thank you to my angels. I most definitely believe in you now because I live in the heart of wine country, where you can throw a grape and hit a domaine.

And in closing, just in case anyone forgot: "I loved my job, I loved my job, I loved my job."

Author Biography

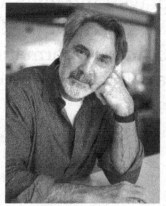

Mark, a New Jersey native (Exit 163), holds an Indus-trial Design degree from The Ohio State University. After years of agency work, his love of acting led him to Hollywood where he appeared in dozens of film, television, and stage productions. Mark also spent his twenty-eight years in Hollywood as an entrepreneur. He started five nonprofit companies, but hold the applause. None were intended to be. He currently lives in the South of France, but hold your pity. He of sound mind and body chose to suffer in the heart of wine country where the locals insist his French isn't so bad—at least that's what he thinks they're saying.

Mark is also an award-winning designer, writer, and director. He has written lots of jokes, several screenplays, and one award-winning short film. *A Cup of Tea on the Commode* is his first memoir. For more information, please visit www.acupofteaonthecommode.org.